Jeppesen's

ADVANCED SPORT DIVER
MANUAL

Richard A. Clinchy III, Editor

Emergency Medical Resources
Plantation, Florida
The American College of Prehospital Medicine
New Orleans, Louisiana

Glen Egstrom, PhD, Associate Editor

Underwater Kinesiology Laboratory
University of California, Los Angeles
Los Angeles, California

Second Edition

with 309 illustrations

Illustrations and artwork by Alan Thompson
Photography by Richard and Nancy Clinchy

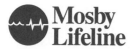

**Mosby
Lifeline**

St. Louis Baltimore Boston Chicago London Philadelphia Sydney Toronto

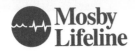
Mosby Lifeline

Publisher: David T. Culverwell
Editor: Richard A. Weimer
Assistant Editor: Julie Bauer
Project Manager: Linda Clarke
Designer: Liz Fett
Photo Credits: Front Cover, Stuart Cummings.

Second Edition

Printed in the United States of America

Mosby–Year Book, Inc.
11830 Westline Industrial Drive
St. Louis, Missouri 63146

Library of Congress Cataloging in Publication Data

Clinchy, Richard A.
    Jeppesen's advanced sport diver manual / Richard A. Clinchy, Glen Egstrom ; illustrations and artwork by Alan Thompson ; photography by Richard and Nancy Clinchy ; with 315 illustrations.—2nd ed.
        p.   cm.
    "A Mosby-Jeppesen product."
    Includes index.
    ISBN 0-8016-9031-5
    1. Diving, Submarine—Handbooks, manuals, etc. I. Egstrom, Glen H. II. Title. III. Title: Advanced sport diver manual.
GV840.S78C52 1993   92-33723
797.2'3—dc20   CIP

93 94 95 96 97 CL/VH 9 8 7 6 5 4 3 2 1

Contributors

Gordon Boivin — Canadian Coast Guard-Rescue Specialist training coordinator and instructor; Officer in Charge, Ocean Rescue Swimmer School, Regional SAR Diving Officer. Vancouver, British Columbia, Canada.

Jeffrey Bozanic — Free-lance diver with specialization in cave and cavern diving. Most recently returned from 5 months as diving supervisor at a research site in Antarctica. Los Angeles, California.

Richard Clinchy — Thirty years' diving experience and a recognized expert both domestically and internationally in emergency medical services. Clinchy is a doctoral candidate in Health Services Management, a Nationally Registered Paramedic, and a Certified Hyperbaric Technologist. Lead Editor and contributor to the *Open Water Sport Diver Manual*. Developer of the Dive/First Responder® training program. Owner of Emergency Medical Resources, Plantation, Florida, and Chairman, The American College of Prehospital Medicine, New Orleans, Louisiana.

Glen Egstrom, PhD — Former Director, Underwater Kinesiology Laboratory, UCLA. Los Angeles, California.

William L. High — Founder of Professional Cylinder Inspectors and a marine fisheries scientist, Bill developed equipment section for the new and as yet unpublished *NOAA Diving Manual*. Seattle, Washington.

Matt McDermott — With an academic background in physiology and over a year's experience with the Ocean Quest operation. He is now part of the Diving Safety Program, University of California at Santa Cruz. Santa Cruz, California.

Daniel Orr — Training Coordinator, Divers Alert Network (DAN), Duke University Medical Center. Contributor to the *NOAA Diving Manual*. Durham, North Carolina.

Robert Rutledge, MD — Anesthesiologist and diving instructor. Education Director of Training Ventures, a dive education firm conducting "top shelf" SCUBA classes and instructor training courses in the Caribbean, with his home in the Caymans as a base. Miami, Florida, and Grand Cayman.

Michael Steidley — SW Regional Sales Manager for SeaQuest, Inc. Mike is also very experienced in free diving and coauthor of *Diving with Dive Computers,* a 1989 text which is quite widely used in the industry. San Diego, California.

Foreword

You have had an opportunity to taste the excitement connected with exploration of the underwater world and can now begin to appreciate why the beauty beneath the seas cannot be described but must be experienced.

In advanced open water training your confidence and basic diving abilities and skills will be improved, no matter what environmental situations you encounter. In addition, you will receive training in boat, beach, and limited visibility diving. Finally, because there are dangers inherent to diving, you will learn how to better deal with emergencies of your own as well as those that might be encountered by your diving companions.

As your training and capabilities improve, never lose sight of the fragility of the underwater realm. In both your diving and your involvement with environmental concerns, help to ensure that the waters that spawned primordial life 3.5 billion years ago will continue to hold beauty and fascination for people as long as our planet exists.

Acknowledgments

Completion of a book of this nature requires the contributions and cooperation of a very large number of people to make it an effort of which those of us coordinating the project can be proud.

First, I must thank the two principal people from Mosby Lifeline, who have been most involved in the completion of this book. Richard Weimer, Senior Editor, has provided immeasurable support, direction, and patient assistance in completing this project. Also, usually in Rick's absence, I have called upon Julie Bauer for her assistance and direction.

To my Assistant Editor, Glen Egstrom, thank you for lending your years of experience and wisdom to this project.

Much of the photography contained herein was done in the Bahamas at Ramada South Ocean, formerly Divi Bahamas Beach Resort & Country Club, Nassau. First, my thanks to Craig J. Burns, Dive Operations Manager, for his cooperation as well as the personnel at Dive South Ocean for their assistance. Members of the Dive South Ocean staff deserving of special mention are Alan and Diana Roberts, Tony McKinney, Errol Lloyd, Andrew Higgs, Sean Lowe, and Wemzel Nichols.

Thanks goes out to Bob Good, owner of Orbit Marine Sports, Pompano Beach, Florida, for his cooperation in completing many of the equipment shots.

Models who agreed to assist and who appear in this book include Nancy Clinchy, Mary Jane Lewis, Matt McDermott, Dalia Jakubauskas, Renee Roberts, Alan Roberts, Marty Knickle, Patrick McKinzey, Tony McKinney, Andrew Higgs, Jennifer Roe, Sean Lowe, Wemzel Nichols, and several others who are not individually identifiable but who appear in group or distance shots.

Several manufacturers have been particularly cooperative in their assistance with this project. Of particular note are:

Ikelite Underwater Systems

Orca Industries

Oceanic Inc.

Boston Whaler

Rite-Bite, Inc.

Submersible Systems

Force Fins

Thanks also to Julie and Keith at Total Chrome, the lab that processes all of my film . . . and even makes some shots better than they started out.

Finally, my wife Nancy served not only as principal model for most of the underwater photography but tolerated the rather arduous ordeal that putting these books together has involved. Sometimes both of us ran short of patience, but we hope the results herein were worth the cost. To Nancy, my thanks and love.

Dick Clinchy, Lead Editor
April 1992

Reviewers, models, and others providing assistance:

Divi Bahamas Beach Resort & Country Club, Nassau

Peter Hughes Diving, Nassau: Peter Hughes, Craig Burns, Harry Ward, Alan and Diana Roberts, Tony McKinney, Errol Lloyd, Andrew Higgs, Sean Lowe, and Wemzel Nichols.

Orbit Marine Sports, Pompano Beach, FL: Bob Good, Marty Knickle-Good, Patrick McKinzey, Mark Reamy.

Divers Den, Ft. Lauderdale, FL: Gary Smith, Dave Smalling, Bernardo Andrade

Jennifer Roe, Baltimore, MD

The Diver's Den, Baltimore, MD: Chaz Kafer

Samuel T. Scott, Arlington, VA

William Cline, Dallas, TX

Tom Griffiths, EdD, Penn State University, State College, PA

Mary Jane Lewis, Dalia Jakubauskas, Stephanie Payne, Renee Roberts, Darrold Garrison, Diana DeNegre, Steve Hansen, Jeff Parker, Matt Stout, Seth Klein

Equipment manufacturers:

Ikelite Underwater Systems, Indianapolis, IN

Oceanic USA, San Leandro, CA

Submersible Systems, Inc., Huntington Beach, CA

Rite Bite Mouthpieces, Inc., Greeley, CO.

Orca Industries, Inc., Toughkenamon, PA

Force Fins, Santa Monica, CA

Quest Marine Video, Mission Viejo, CA

Photography: Dick & Nancy Clinchy, Jeff Bozanic, Matt McDermott, J. Gale Livers, Mary Brooks, Steve Lucas, Julie Bauer

Artwork: Allan Thompson

Contents

1 Equipment Techniques

At the conclusion of this chapter, you should be able to:

1. Properly explain the procedure for cleaning the lens of a mask to prevent fogging.
2. Explain how you describe to another diver how to determine whether a purge valve in the mask is working properly prior to starting a dive.
3. Name the four alternative methods of vision correction with diving masks.
4. Tell what safety feature should be in place on a snorkel tube.
5. Tell how often proper weighting and buoyancy should be checked.
6. State how often tanks should be both visually inspected and hydrostatically tested.
7. State how often your regulator should be serviced and under what conditions service may be needed more frequently.
8. Explain how you should sharpen your knife when it becomes dull and why.
9. State the accuracy of most depth gauges.
10. Summarize the nine basic rules of computer diving.

KEY TERMS

Ozone	Mold splashings	Cummerbund (Cummerband)
Under-weighting	Weight clips	
Unbalanced	Balanced	Hose protectors
Dynamic dive monitor	Over-weighting	

Scuba diving is an equipment-intensive sport. It is impossible to dive without it; the mask, snorkel, fins, buoyancy compensator, cylinder, regulator, gauges, and other equipment items are the diver's underwater life support system. No matter how experienced a diver may be, dives should be made with complete and appropriate equipment. A diver is not safe simply because he or she can breathe underwater. Under optimum conditions, in shallow water, it may be possible to make

1

some dives with minimum equipment, but to be comfortable and safe, the diver needs to prepare for the unexpected.

All the equipment in the world will not make a diver safe unless it is of excellent quality. Fortunately, gone are the days of diving with the two-hose regulator without nonreturn valves; a narrow, corrugated snorkel; flimsy fins; tank harnesses made of webbing; low visibility masks; and other, similar equipment. Today, equipment improvements as well as new equipment designs appear so frequently that the diver has ample opportunity to use the most modern diving equipment available.

Even the finest diving equipment is not maintenance free. Divers, like many people in other activities, may assume that equipment should simply work correctly, and they are often quick to blame others for any malfunction. However, equipment failure is rarely a problem, because today's equipment is carefully manufactured, refined, and dependable. Most diving accidents can be traced to human error, which includes poor equipment maintenance, equipment misuse, lack of equipment-related skills, and misunderstanding of equipment.

The situations you encounter as an advanced diver require that you have more understanding and skills than you may have had as an open water diver. This is particularly true in areas such as how your equipment functions, any modifications or adjustments needed for different situations, and other potential problems. When you master your equipment, your advanced diving career becomes filled with pleasurable and memorable rather than hair-raising underwater experiences.

Diving Equipment in General

Diving equipment, as you know, can be subdivided into several categories: equipment that helps vision, equipment that enables movement, equipment that protects from the environment, life-sustaining equipment such as regulators and tanks, buoyancy control equipment, and information equipment.

Unless you can see, there is virtually no reason to dive, so the mask becomes the first essential piece of equipment. Next, the snorkel allows you to breathe comfortably at the surface. The combination of regulator and tank provide the ability to breathe comfortably at depth. The fins provide the propulsion needed to move easily through the water. All this allows you to stay underwater for extended periods. However, extended stays underwater can produce discomfort, so you may need dive skins, a wet suit, or a dry suit for environmental protection. When suits enter the picture you become more positively buoyant. To offset this, you need a weight belt and some kind of buoyancy compensator. The buoyancy compensator allows you to adjust for the decrease in the suit's buoyancy when you dive at depth.

To stay at depths comfortably for extended periods requires a cylinder and regulator and the equipment to attach them to your body. Longer bottom times bring up another problem—extended exposure to pressure. To avoid any difficulties because of this, you need to be equipped with information regarding your dive. Information equipment tells you how long you have been down, how deep you are, how near to the need for decompression you are, and what direction you are going.

This basic equipment is fundamental for prudent scuba diving; to dive with anything less is unwise. This material is intended to give you information beyond what you received in open water diver training on equipment fit and maintenance. Selection of equipment will be reviewed because you may want to replace or add equipment for certain advanced diving activities.

MASK, SNORKEL, AND FINS

During your open water training and from your subsequent diving experiences, you received an understanding of the most basic diving tools—the mask, snorkel, and fins. There are a few pointers, however, that can help you to use these tools more effectively and to avoid future problems.

Mask Fit

Mask fit is extremely important. Leakage or discomfort occurs when your mask does not fit properly. To avoid both problems, be sure that the mask, when placed lightly against your face, touches everywhere and that the seal provides a comfortable, uniform contact with your face. This is important when you wear the mask for long periods, because the seal creates pressure that, in turn, can cause discomfort if the mask is improperly fitted. Adjust the strap so the mask fits evenly on your face. The split-strap or broad-coverage headband should fit uniformly on the crown of your head as shown in Figs. 1-1 and 1-2. The mask should be tight enough to stay on, but not tight enough to cause an uncomfortable squeeze. As manufacturers continue to improve mask design and materials, it becomes easier for the scuba diver to find a mask that fits comfortably, does not leak, and accomplishes both tasks in such a way that the mask itself goes relatively unnoticed by the diver once in place.

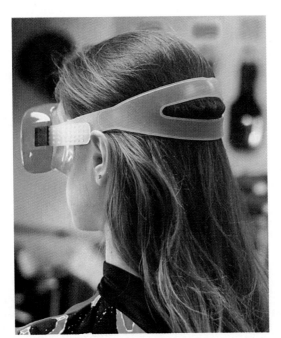

Fig. 1-1 *Standard mask strap placement. (Courtesy of Julie Bauer.)*

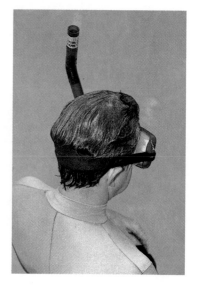

Fig. 1-2 Broad-coverage type of mask securing band.

Mask Maintenance

The most frequent mask problems include fogging, slipping straps, and rotting. The best solution to lens fogging is prevention. This includes cleaning the mask with toothpaste, a mild kitchen cleanser, or the cleaner provided with the mask at time of purchase. This is done before you use the mask for the first time in order to remove the silicone the manufacturer places on the mask to protect it during shipping and to assure that the lens is cleaned of any other film or substance that might increase fogging. You will need to clean your mask periodically to remove chemicals, such as sun screen, makeup, and preservatives, from the face plate.

Immediately before your dive, use commercially available chemical wetting agents or liquid dishwashing soap for defogging. Remember, rinse the inside of the mask thoroughly after applying defogger so that none of the chemical will accidentally run into your eyes. Wetting agents tend to be a little more acceptable aesthetically, but in the absence of wetting agents, saliva might work.

Although black rubber masks are seen less frequently now than in past years, some divers still use them. The best way to prevent black rubber masks from rotting is to coat the rubber parts of the mask, except the strap, with silicone or some other form of rubber preservative. The mask strap should not be lubricated because silicone is slippery and could cause the strap to slip unexpectedly. This protective measure on the other rubber parts of the mask prevents ozone from reaching the material and keeps it supple and durable.

Silicone masks do not need to be protected with silicone or any other substance; they simply need to be kept clean and should be rinsed in fresh water after each dive. However, silicone masks should never be placed touching any black rubber equipment, as the silicone will become discolored by such contact.

Breakage of the retainer buckles, strap, lens, and frame can be prevented by inspecting the mask and carefully placing it in your gear bag. If your mask has any metal parts, watch for corrosion, as well. If your mask has metal buckles, keep the

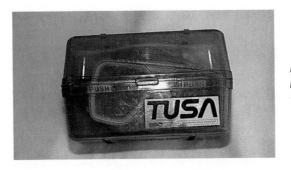

Fig. 1-3 *Use the carrying case supplied with your mask before putting in your gear bag.*

buckles clean by washing them in fresh water after each use. Most modern masks are purchased with a reusable plastic carrying case (Fig. 1-3). Risk of lens breakage can be significantly reduced by placing your mask back in this case before putting it in your gear bag. It is not totally possible to prevent the strap and lens from breaking, but you can replace these parts easily in quality masks.

If your mask has a purge valve, check its function before you dive by inhaling to hold the mask on your face and exhaling to force air out as you hold the mask firmly on your face with your hands. If the valve is stuck open, the mask will not stay on your face when you inhale, and if it is stuck shut, you will not be able to exhale through your nose. Occasionally, purge valves have a small portion that becomes inverted, making proper operation of the valve impossible. This is easily corrected by simply prying this portion back into position to make the valve work properly. If your mask fits properly and water seeps into your mask during a dive, the purge valve may have become weak. In this case, replace the valve.

Men with beards and moustaches sometimes find that it is more difficult to maintain a mask seal because of the facial hair—remember your instructor during your open water course telling you to make sure all the hair was out of the mask seal? A trick that has worked fairly well to solve this problem has been the use of petroleum jelly or a similar substance. Simply smear petroleum jelly into the portion of the moustache that will contact the mask seal, flatten the hair out in the direction that it normally grows, and put on the mask. After the dive, remember to clean the mask skirt well to remove the petroleum jelly.

Should you have vision difficulties, you should give consideration to prescription lenses for your mask or wearing contact lenses. There are several alternatives available to you:

1. Some mask manufacturers can supply lenses that closely approximate the prescription supplied by your optometrist or ophthalmologist. These lenses are easily installed by your dive store professional or may be installed yourself.
2. Opticians, particularly in communities where diving is popular, have the capability to grind lenses specifically suited to your personal prescription and adjusted for the optic influence of water.
3. A third alternative utilizing mask lenses is the "glue-on" corrective lens. Uti-

lizing acrylic cement, a lens with the appropriate correction for your vision is cemented to the flat glass lens of the diving mask.

4. A final option is the wire holder that can be fitted inside a mask to hold conventional glasses, minus the temples, inside the mask.

Regardless of the approach utilized, there is no reason why you should not dive with appropriate correction for any vision defect you may have.

Both wide-angle masks and translucent silicon masks make your diving experiences appear "brighter." Plus, wide-angle masks give the diver improved peripheral vision.

However, if you expect to be shooting a lot of underwater video or using a housed camera, it will probably be easier for you to see clearly what is in the viewfinder of your camera if you use a mask with an opaque mask skirt (preferably black). If that is the case, maybe two masks should be in the diver's equipment bag—one that is wide-angle or translucent for routine diving, and a second mask that is black or opaque for underwater photography or video.

Snorkel Fit

The snorkel should be adjusted so as you look straight down, the snorkel is as nearly vertical as possible. (See Fig. 1-4.)

Flexibility of the snorkel barrel should take into consideration the environment in which you will be diving. If you are going to be doing river diving, diving in overhead environments, or using the snorkel primarily to supplement scuba, a flexible snorkel is probably most appropriate.

The mouthpiece should not press too hard on either your upper or lower gums, as this can irritate your mouth. If the mouthpiece is uncomfortable, you can sand the edges, trim it with scissors, or, in some cases, replace the mouthpiece. Several commercially available snorkels have mouthpieces that are adjustable utilizing a swivel-type connection to the snorkel barrel so they will fit parallel to the gum line for comfort.

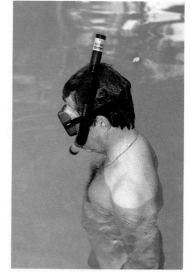

Fig. 1-4 *Snorkel placement places the snorkel in a position where it will be nearly vertical when you look straight down.*

A new variety of mouthpiece, useful for both snorkels and scuba regulator mouthpieces, has been designed by a dentist to allow for the natural position of the jaw and teeth, fit in the mouth more securely, and essentially eliminate jaw fatigue. The dive store that handles these mouthpieces can easily determine which of the three available fits are appropriate and will have a mouthpiece on hand to modify your snorkel or regulator (Fig. 1-5). Regardless of how you accomplish it, make sure you get a mouthpiece for your snorkel that is comfortable and fits well.

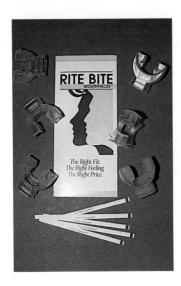

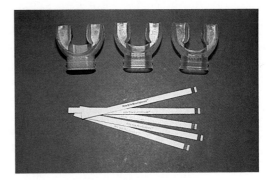

Fig. 1-5 *A new variety of mouthpiece allowing maximum fit and comfort for snorkels and regulators. (Courtesy of Rite Bite Mouthpieces, Inc.)*

Snorkel Maintenance

The greatest snorkel problems come primarily from wear. To prevent deterioration from ozone, keep a black rubber snorkel lubricated with a rubber preservative such as silicone. Silicone snorkels require little maintenance to prevent deterioration. Regularly wash the snorkel with water and clean it once in a while with a mouthwash, disinfectant, or soap. Do not forget to check the snorkel keeper for wear and replace it whenever wear is noticed. Most newer snorkels are equipped with devices to attach them to mask straps, which are quite rigid and less subject to wear than the older "butterfly" type snorkel keepers.

The longer the snorkel, the greater the breathing resistance. If this is a problem you encounter, you can shorten the snorkel. Just make sure the end is still above the surface of the water when you use it. You should always replace the brightly colored band by attaching bright tape to the top of the tube. If your snorkel did not come with this band, be sure to use bright-colored tape, so you will be easier to see in the water when snorkeling.

Fin Fit

Your fins should fit tight enough so they do not slide on your feet, but at the same time, they should be loose enough so you do not experience cramps. If you have adjustable straps, set them snugly enough so they hold, but not so tight as to make

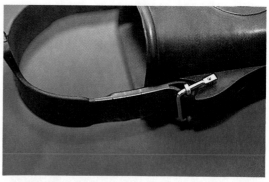

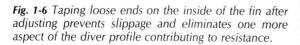

Fig. 1-6 Taping loose ends on the inside of the fin after adjusting prevents slippage and eliminates one more aspect of the diver profile contributing to resistance.

the toes rub against the end of the foot pockets. Turn the straps so they are threaded through the buckle system with the loose ends on the inside. (See Fig. 1-6.) If you do not anticipate any need to adjust fin fit, wrap the loose ends with black electrical tape so they are secure.

Some divers like to lubricate the foot pockets with silicone spray, WD40, Armorall, or a similar product to make it easier to slip the foot or bootie into the foot pocket. It is important not to allow any of that lubricant onto the fin straps or there may be a risk of slippage while diving.

Fins sometimes come from the manufacturer with small pieces of rubber or silicone, called *mold splashings,* protruding from drain holes and foot pockets. Carefully trim these off with a sharp, thin knife or razor so they do not interfere with how the fins fit.

Fin Maintenance

A limited number of things can go wrong with fins. Adjustable straps may break or heel pockets of full-foot fins may break through. When a heel pocket breaks, you can no longer use the fins; however, when a strap breaks, you can replace it. It is a good practice to carry, in your dive bag or "goody" box, extra fin straps that fit your fins. It is a lot cheaper to purchase a couple of extra fin straps than to have an entire dive trip ruined by something as simple as a broken fin strap. You should watch for wear and check the straps regularly. If you notice wear marks, replace the straps before they break. With fewer and fewer rubber fins in use today and as more silicone is utilized, these problems are diminishing, but nevertheless, straps are still an area that can wear and fail.

Buckles, if they are metal, sometimes separate and become loose, so tap the ends with a hammer and nail set to flatten and secure them. Another thing to look for on metal fin parts is corrosion both on the buckle and pin mechanism. If your fins have metal buckles, it is a good idea to carry an extra buckle in your repair kit along with the fin straps. More modern fin buckles are made of noncorrosive materials and are designed to avoid the failure problems often associated with older fin designs (Fig. 1-7).

Fin pockets filled with sand and debris are an inconvenience. You can minimize this problem by drilling holes into the top sole of the foot pockets. The holes should be no larger than one-fourth inch to be effective.

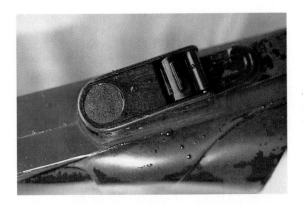

Fig. 1-7 Modern fin buckle designs avoid many of the maintenance problems once associated with fin buckles.

One other aspect of fin maintenance involves marking. It is a good idea, especially if you plan to do much boat diving, to mark your name or some other identifying mark on your fins so they will not be confused with another diver's fins. Any office supply store can provide you with a marking device that utilizes a quick-drying paint that will easily adhere to any fin material and will wear very well over time.

WEIGHT BELT

Adjustments

Some buoyancy compensators (BC) have integral weighting systems that are theoretically positioned to provide the diver with the most comfortable attitude (position) in the water. These built-in systems also provide a mechanism for ditching the weights in an emergency. The only significant adjustment with such weight systems is amount of weight. It is a good practice to check weighting each time you dive to be certain that you are neither over-weighted nor under-weighted. Over-weighting adds risk to your diving, requires greater amounts of air in your BC to maintain a depth, and thereby increases your drag in the water. Under-weighting forces the diver to work harder to stay at depth with increased fatigue and air consumption.

The type of weighting system typically used is the weight belt, or external weighting system. Two considerations for the external weights are placement of weight and type of buckle. The weights should be set just slightly forward of the center of the hips, as shown in Fig. 1-8. This lets you rest facing forward more easily and reduces, to a great extent, the sensation of the tank and backpack pulling you backward. The advantage of the weight belt is that its position can be altered as you dive. Ideally, the position of the weight belt is one that makes you feel most comfortable and allows you to maintain as nearly a level position as possible in the water. The position of your weight belt needs to be coordinated with the position of your tank on each dive as the tank, depending upon type and amount of air remaining, will also influence your attitude in the water.

When using conventional lead weights and a standard weight belt, you need to prevent weights from sliding off your belt when putting the belt on or taking it off.

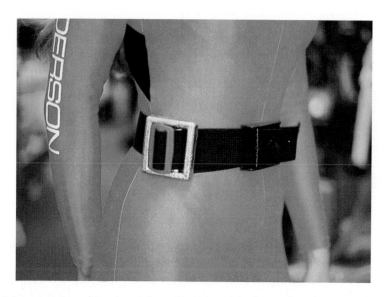

Fig. 1-8 *When wearing external weights, place them just forward of the center of the hips. (Courtesy of Julie Bauer).*

Also, weights need to be stabilized so they will not slide around when the belt is in place. Use either weight clips (Fig. 1-9) or twist the belt once after it has been placed through one of the slots and then slip the strap through the other slot (Fig. 1-10). This procedure should be followed with at least the first and last weight on your belt. Another technique that may be used to secure multiple weights is the stacking of weights. This method not only allows for securing weights but also aids in establishing a center of gravity that the diver may find most comfortable for the diving situation. Another method favored by some divers is to drive a small nail or screw through the belt material into the soft lead weight. This technique secures the weight's location fairly reliably but makes it a little more cumbersome to quickly change weights. Some recent innovations in weight belt design (see Fig. 1-11) utilize pockets in a mesh, subdivided, zippered pouch along the weight belt. This prevents the weights from shifting position and enables you to modify weight when changing protective suits.

Whatever the design of the weight-carrying device, the belt must have a quick-release buckle or quick-release system. Although some belts may have wire frame or metal buckles, most weight belt buckles today are manufactured from a variety of thermoplastics. Also, the placement of the buckle on your weight belt should be distinctive from all other buckles on your equipment and typically oriented opposite your BC buckle, typically a right-hand release is appropriate. This helps both you and your buddy easily distinguish the weight belt buckle in the event of an emergency requiring the ditching of the weight belt. Especially when wearing a compressible wet suit, it is important to periodically check the position of your weight belt buckle. As the wet suit material compresses, the belt may shift position

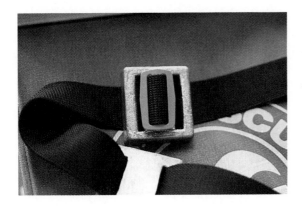

Fig. 1-9 *Weight clips will prevent conventional weights from slipping or falling off the belt when it is either put on or taken off. (Courtesy of Julie Bauer.)*

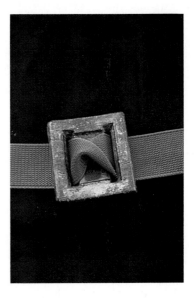

Fig. 1-10 *Twisting the belt as it is passed through the first and last weight on your buckle will prevent slippage.*

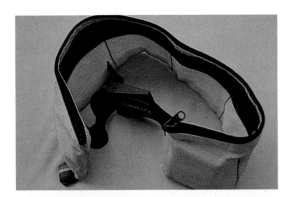

Fig. 1-11 *Some belt designs utilize a mesh, subdivided pouch to handle weights and prevent slippage.*

and move into a potentially unsafe location. You need only slip your hand to your waist and feel for the weight belt buckle to be sure it is still accessible. If it has shifted position, simply slip it around to where both you and your buddy can easily have access to it in an emergency (Fig. 1-12).

Always preparing for an emergency, one skill that you should practice on a regular basis is the ditching of your weight belt. How significant a factor is this in diving accidents? In a review of the major accident reports published over the last several years, over 80% of divers who lost their lives were still wearing their weight belts. In a real emergency, ditching the weight belt can be your "elevator" to the surface. Make sure that your weight belt is easily accessible and uncomplicated to ditch. Positive ditching of the weight belt is a critical skill that cannot be overpracticed. The belt must be free to drop when released. Therefore, in practicing this skill, pull it away from your body and do not have any obstruction in the droppath of the belt. If you are in a marginal situation, positive buoyancy is great insurance. At any time you need to ditch your weight belt in an emergency, drop anything in your hands and use both hands to ditch your weight belt. No "treasure" or piece of diving equipment is worth your life!

Today, lead shot–filled belts with a velcro attachment to the weight belt are a more comfortable compliant alternative to the solid lead weights that have been used for years in diving (Fig. 1-13). With the evolution of shot-filled weight belts, ankle weights have also gained in popularity for those who have difficulty maintaining a horizontal attitude due to buoyancy in the legs. Whatever type of weight system utilized, be completely familiar with your system and be as familiar with your buddy's system as you are with your own!

Maintenance

If your weight belt is equipped with a metal or wire frame release, make certain that they are free of corrosion and easily released in an emergency. If you are using a thermoplastic weight belt buckle, check it before every dive to be certain the buckle has not cracked. The end of the weight belt strap should be cut so no more than 6 inches of belt protrudes from the buckle when the belt is donned with

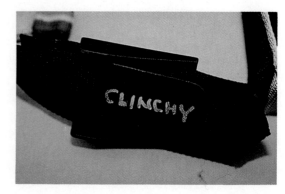

Fig. 1-12 *The weight belt buckle should be situated so that it is easily distinguished and opposite other buckles on your equipment.*

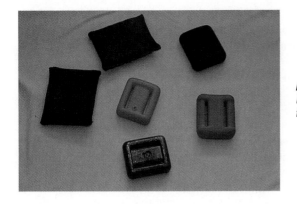

Fig. 1-13 *A variety of weights are available today including shot-filled weight bags that tend to be more comfortable than conventional weights.*

weights and protective suit. The nylon strap ends should be free of any frayed material. This can be accomplished by heating the material with an open flame after it has been cut to length. The heat seals and congeals the end of the fibers. Applying of a light coat of wet suit cement to the belt end will assure that the belt will not fray if the material begins to unravel. Application of liquid vinyl, which can be found in most hardware stores, is another approach to prevent fraying of the belt end.

BUOYANCY COMPENSATORS

As your experience in diving expands, you will come to recognize that there are a myriad of choices when it comes to BCs. The variety ranges from the smaller front mounted ("horse-collar") devices to back-mounted BCs, to the jacket style BC, to the BC that has integral weights. All have their relative advantages but none should become a crutch for the scuba diver.

The BC needs to be selected based on the amount of weight utilized by the scuba diver. The primary objective among environmentally and safety concerned divers today is to wear as little weight as possible. This reduces the risk of overweight damage to the environment, reduces the amount of air required in a BC to remain neutrally buoyant, and thereby reduces the amount of effort required by the scuba diver to complete a dive. Let's review just a little of what the concept of neutral buoyancy entails.

At the end of a dive with at least 500 psi in your tank, if you can hang at the 10-foot depth without any air in your BC, then you are neutrally buoyant. If you must add air to your BC, then you are too heavy. How much difference does this all make in your diving? A great deal. First, if you are over-weighted, you need to put more air in your BC to remain neutral. Regardless of the type of BC utilized, this will put you into a head high attitude in the water, requiring more energy on the part of the diver to move through the water. Additionally, as you are pitched into this head-high attitude, your fins are put in a lower position relative to your body, making it more likely that they will do damage to the environment. So, before looking at the specific types and features of BCs, let's try to become less dependent upon them for retention of neutral buoyancy and instead, attain that state by reduction of weight. For too long, the attitude has been to somewhat overweight, making it easier to get down, and then compensate for the over-weighting with the BC. The practice tends to be unsafe and is certainly not environmentally responsible.

First, from a safety standpoint, the BC should be capable of keeping a scuba diver's head above the surface of the water when inflated at the surface. Since the adult head weighs between 7.5 and 10 kilograms (16.5 to 22 pounds), it becomes obvious that it does not take a massive amount of air to displace that weight and keep the head above water. Understanding that aspect of buoyancy and combining that knowledge with proper weighting, the scuba diver should end up with a device, regardless of design, most aptly suited to buoyancy control needs. A good rule of thumb is that a BC's buoyant lift *must* equal or exceed the amount of weight worn.

The horse-collar design was the earliest of the diving BCs and is still utilized by some divers. The advantage of this design is its relative simplicity and the versatility that such a BC offers in that it is useful for both skin and scuba diving. Inflation mechanisms on these devices vary from oral inflation, to low-pressure inflation from the scuba tank, to a British design that has a built-in moderate volume cylinder into which air from the scuba tank is transferred for buoyancy-control purposes. Such a device adds whatever buoyancy might be needed to adjust for buoyancy losses at depth as well as providing needed buoyancy to keep the head above the surface of the water for safety purposes. Two disadvantages of this type of BC include the need for a separate backpack for tank mounting as contrasted to the integral backpack that is a part of most other BCs. Also, it should be noted that nearly all dive operators supply bare tanks and do not have backpacks available. Secondly, this type of BC usually requires the use of a crotch strap that necessitates particular caution in putting the weight belt on last so ditching the weight belt is not in any way impeded by other equipment.

The jacket-style BC is probably the most popular of all devices currently used (see Figs. 1-14 and 1-15). This style combines attractive styling, integral backpack, ease of inflation from a low-pressure hose, and back-up oral inflation. In the better-designed jacket-style BCs, the buoyancy air is distributed under the arms and to the waist area. Such buoyancy lift is useful for offsetting losses of buoyancy at depth without shifting the diver's center of gravity relative to neutral buoyancy. Features that make some of these BCs superior include adequate self-draining pockets for storage of any equipment, tables, or other items taken along on a dive, but the diver should recognize that such pockets tend to add to drag. A velcro fastening cummerbund that secures the BC in position and maintains its location on the diver relative to center of gravity is another good feature. On the left side of the BC should be an inflator hose that incorporates both an oral inflator valve, manual deflator mechanism, and a valve allowing use of low-pressure tank air to inflate the BC. Recently, an addition to the low-pressure inflator hose has been an alternate second stage regulator that the diver can utilize in the event of the need for air sharing or failure of the primary second stage. Low-profile jacket style BCs have quick release buckles just below the shoulders on the front allowing quick ditching

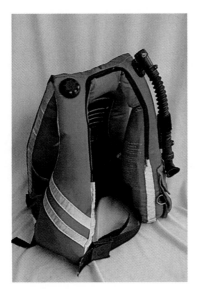

Fig. 1-14 Older jacket-style BC. Notice the location of the buoyancy envelope or bubble.

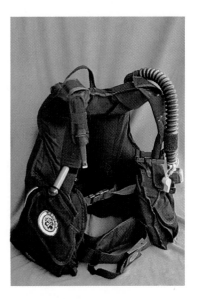

Fig. 1-15 The jacket-style BC of a more modern design. The envelope/bubble is under the arms and at the waist and the BC is equipped with quick-release buckles for rapid ditching of the device in an emergency.

of the BC in an emergency. Older style jacket BCs generally have their air bag/bladder extending up to and over the shoulder, which restricts motion and does not allow for ditching as quickly as the devices equipped with the quick-release buckles. Finally, there should be an air dump valve (rapid exhaust) that is located at the highest point in the air pocket or bubble established by the inflated BC. Such a valve allows for rapid dumping of air in the event of an over-inflation emergency or if the need to rapidly deflate the BC should ever arise, such as a rescue. Also, as you become more experienced as a diver, the rapid exhaust can be used for regular deflation to control buoyancy.

The third general type of BC is the buoyancy control pack or back mounted BC, which wraps around the tank to the rear of the diver. These BCs require more training than others since their inflation tends to push the diver into a face-down position, necessitating practice to maintain oneself in a proper position both at depth and on the surface.

The type of BC that is appropriate for the diving you anticipate will largely dictate your choice. If you want a BC that you can utilize equally well in the skin diving and scuba diving environment then the well-designed horse-collar BC is appropriate. If you anticipate learning skills such as cave, cavern, or penetration wreck diving then consideration should be given to a BC that will present the most compact profile when you are wearing it. The average scuba diver whose diving may employ various types of exposure suits should make certain that the type of BC selected has maximum capability to adjust size so the BC will not restrict movement when wearing a thick wet suit or dry suit.

Fit

Before you purchase a BC, you should try on a variety of models while wearing the exposure protection you intend to use diving. This helps to ensure proper fit and allows you to determine the comfort of the device. The areas that are most important are the upper chest, the upper waist, and the torso length. With the BC in place, inflate the bladder fully and be certain that the bubble of the bladder expands away from the body harnessing. If the bladder expands inward toward the body, it may severely restrict your breathing capability in an emergency and is not an appropriate BC for you to consider. Straps should be adjusted on the front mounted BC with it fully inflated to keep the vest from riding up and creating discomfort in the neck area and crotch. A properly attached and adjusted crotch strap is the only effective way to keep the inflated BC bladder down in the front mounted, horse collar type BC. If the BC you are considering has a strap at the waist, you should easily be able to open and close it with one hand. This will assure that you will easily be able to resecure an errant BC or ditch the device in an emergency with as little difficulty as possible. Almost all buckles on newer BCs are one-hand operated, quick-release buckles that allow easily removing the BC in an emergency. Most of the straps used to adjust the waist dimensions of the BCs are velcro closures on modern devices. It is important to carefully maintain all velcro closures to assure that they are free of debris to ensure continued reliable closure.

The backpack of the BC needs to be properly adjusted for fit as well. Correct adjustment keeps the unit from riding up off your back during inflation of the BC. Be sure the shoulder and waist straps are properly adjusted and fit snugly. To prevent confusion, the backpack and/or BC buckle should have the release oriented opposite to the weight belt release. For most right-handed people this means a left-handed release for the BC or backpack and a right-handed release for the weight belt. If you are left hand dominant, it may be better to reverse this pattern since you should be capable of easily releasing the weight belt buckle single-handedly and have both hands available for ditching the weight belt.

BC jackets need less adjustment, except for the front buckles, which should fasten near the middle of the waist (Fig. 1-16). A good fit is most important. The BC should fit snugly, yet still allow room for inflation. In some poorly designed jacket BCs, this is virtually impossible as they become uncomfortably tight when inflated. That is why it is particularly important to try on the BC you are considering and check it for fit and comfort both inflated and deflated.

Following purchase of your BC and adjustment of all straps and buckles, the strap material should be trimmed with any ends heated to prevent fraying. An electric soldering iron can be used to trim and heat treat the material in a single operation.

Once all the basic straps and buckles are adjusted, check the placement of pockets (many BCs have removable pockets). Check the length of the BC inflator hose and if it does not feel comfortable replace it with an appropriate length hose. Make sure that there are appropriate attachments or "keepers" on the BC to manage the octopus hose, console or computer hose, or any other device or equipment that will routinely be carried while diving. With all such attachments and equipment you should consider how you will be "streamlined" while in the water—keep drag in mind at any time you add any equipment to your standard diving gear.

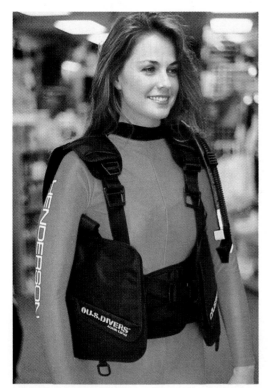

Fig. 1-16 *The wraparound BC adjusted for fit. (Courtesy of Julie Bauer.)*

Most of the newer BCs have integrated backpacks and many are of the softer, contoured variety. These make wearing of a backpack far more comfortable and limit the pressure points on various parts of the diver's back that used to be common with the older, hard backpacks.

Maintenance

BCs are susceptible to wear and tear, primarily because they extend outward from your body even when deflated. The most troublesome wear is caused by punctures or abrasions, but proper care and handling can prevent excess wear on this valuable piece of diving equipment.

Salt water can damage both the exterior and interior of a BC. Since some water leaks in when the dump valve, or oral inflator/deflator valve is operated, you must rinse the interior of the BC after every dive. The best way to do this is to fill the BC with air and flood the interior with warm, fresh water. Then, move the vest from side to side and top to bottom and, finally, open the valve to let the water completely drain out. Contamination in the dump valve can prevent it from sealing properly and cause it to leak. This problem can be avoided by rinsing the valve with fresh, clean water. As a final step, inflate the BC and hang it up so residual moisture can drain into the oral inflation-deflation hose.

CO_2 cartridges used to be a common "safety" addition to the BC, but with inadvertent firings resulting in sudden excessive buoyancy and the corrosion problems frequently associated with the cartridges modern scuba has largely done away with the CO_2 cartridge as a supplement to the BC. If you do choose to use CO_2 cartridges, remember to rinse out the CO_2 mechanism at the same time the BC is rinsed with clean, fresh water. To do this, remove the CO_2 cartridge and flush out the threaded CO_2 mount with fresh water from inside the BC as well as from outside. After the BC has dried, use a water-soluble lubricant when reinstalling the cartridge if the installation will be metal to metal and a silicone lubricant if the CO_2 cartridge mount is plastic. Before every dive you should check the cartridge and firing mechanism for possible corrosion or malfunction. During every dive when using CO_2 cartridges, be particularly cautious to avoid accidental discharge of the cartridge as the resultant rapid increase in buoyancy could lead to serious injury. When diving in any form of overhead environment (i.e., under ice, caves and caverns, and penetration wreck dives) it is more advisable to remove the CO_2 cartridge than to keep it installed—it presents a greater risk than the benefit of emergency buoyancy offered by CO_2.

TANKS

Adjustment

Most backpacks are an integral part of the BC, as shown in Fig. 1-17. When you attach the tank to the backpack, it is important to check the height of the tank and be certain that the mechanism that fastens the tank to the backpack is secure. Many BCs have a strap at the top which will help you to adjust the tank to the proper height. To double check the appropriate height of the tank in the backpack, tip your head back with the backpack in place. Your head should not touch the tank

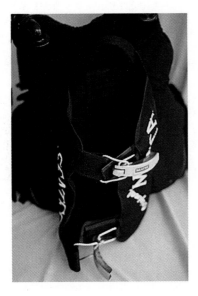

Fig. 1-17 This BC has the backpack incorporated as part of the BC structure.

valve in this position. If it does, lower your tank in the backpack to a level where your head does not make contact with the tank valve when your head is tipped back. If using nylon and web belts to secure the tank, try to wet them before securing the tank and periodically check them for security as they do require attention. After the tank has been properly secured to the backpack, pick up the backpack from the deck with tank attached and shake it gently to check that it is securely fastened (Fig. 1-18).

When you don the tank and backpack, lift them high on your back and make sure the shoulder straps are tight enough to hold the tank and backpack securely in place. At the same time be certain that your arms are free to move sufficiently. Finally, pull the waist strap or cummerbund so it is snug and secure.

Fig. 1-18 The top of the backpack should be at the same level as the top of the tank where it narrows.

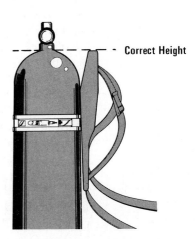

Correct Height

Provided you will be using the same exposure suit at all times, your backpack can be adjusted permanently with extra webbing trimmed in the same manner as the weight belt. If you will be using varying weights of exposure suit, make your "permanent" backpack adjustments with the bulkiest of your exposure suits donned. Once you have all your backpack straps adjusted for length, secure the waist strap with its release oriented opposite that of your weight belt, as previously discussed. Once all of these strap adjustments are made you can then trim away all excess strap material.

Backpack maintenance includes maintaining the buckles and straps just as you do those on the weight belt. Whether you use heat to treat strap ends or choose to tape them, you need to check all strap ends periodically for fraying and the straps themselves for deterioration and the need of replacement. Your dive store professional should have a ready supply of repair and replacement parts or should be capable of easily securing them on relatively short notice.

Maintenance

The *Open Water Sport Diver Manual* contains an extensive discussion regarding scuba tanks and their care but a few additional items are worthy of mention.

Tanks should be visually inspected by a reputable dive store with personnel trained in visual inspection at least once a year and any time there is obvious or suspected damage or doubt in your mind of the tank's safety or integrity such as the presence of corrosion, cuts, gouges, and pits. It is recommended that rental cylinders or those undergoing heavy use be inspected more frequently, perhaps as often as once every 3 months. A tank should also be inspected any time the air has an odor or taste, and each time it is completely emptied on a dive. Water inside a tank can quickly destroy it.

The U.S. Department of Transportation requires tanks to be hydrostatically tested every 5 years. You should also have your tanks tested any time you see obvious damage. Aluminum cylinders that have been exposed to temperatures in excess of 305° F (176° C), should be condemned. If you feel that a tank has been exposed to temperatures nearly this high, have the tank hydrostatically tested—it may be condemned after failing the test. Do not use catalyst paint strippers and never modify the finish on a tank yourself. The only things that a diver should have on a tank other than the factory finish might be a sticker or decal. Failure to heed this advice regarding tank safety and maintenance may result in a ruptured tank, which could lead to serious injury. Several other tank problems, like those shown in Fig. 1-19, also can occur.

The probability of fresh water damage that would remove a tank from service is rare. The types of damage that can cause a tank to deteriorate over a period of time can usually be avoided by thoroughly rinsing the tank's exterior with clean, fresh water after each use. Continual exposure to salt water requires this rinsing process to avoid structural tank damage.

When using tank boots, mesh tank protectors, and tank covers, it is especially important that these be removed and rinsed separately from the tank and allowed to thoroughly dry separately before replacing them on the tank.

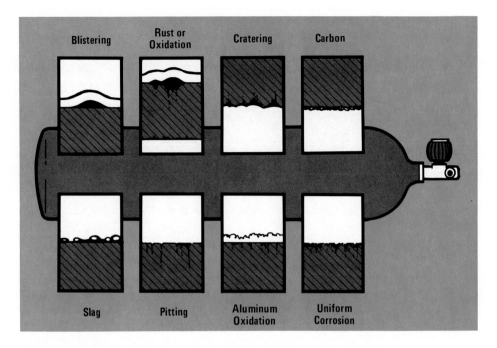

Fig. 1-19 *Examples of the types of other tank problems that may damage either steel or aluminum cylinders.*

Technology is rapidly evolving in the area of scuba tanks and the future of diving offers stronger tank materials, more compact tanks, and a greater air supply. In Europe, the DIN fitting, which allows significantly higher tank pressures, has been commonplace for many years. This technology has now come to the United States Recreational scuba community, making available a 100-cubic foot tank that is no larger than the standard 80-foot tank. The future for high-volume, high-pressure tanks is bright and the day will probably come in the future that a single tank will contain adequate air for the average scuba diver to make two full-length dives on a single tank of air.

REGULATOR

Selection

Single hose regulators are manufactured primarily in two basic designs. Both first and second stages can be either balanced or unbalanced. Unbalanced regulators have a relative increase in breathing resistance at decreased tank pressures (300 to 600 psi), which causes a difference in how well the first stage valve opens and closes. Theoretically, there is more effort to breathe at the end of a dive than at the beginning of the dive relative to opening the first stage valve during inhalation.

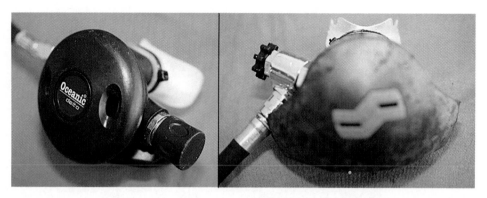

Fig. 1-20 *Second stage adjustment to modify breathing resistance during the dive.*

However, studies performed at the U.S. Navy Experimental Diving Unit demonstrated that the differences between balanced and unbalanced regulators at recreational diving depths are relatively insignificant, so this aspect of regulator design should not be paramount in your choice of regulator. The unbalanced regulator is usually simpler and requires less frequent maintenance.

The key to appropriate regulator selection should be quality of function. Try a wide variety of rental regulators until you find one with which you are comfortable. In general, if you want dependable, smooth regulator operation and intend to use the equipment frequently, choose the high-end balanced regulator. This design functions with minimum breathing effort and at maximum efficiency, providing little breathing resistance at all tank pressures (Fig. 1-20).

Other features that should be considered are regulators with user-adjustable flow at the second stage. These regulators can be regulated while diving to maintain a degree of breathing ease consistent with the individual diver's needs. Some second stages also provide a device that humidifies the air you breathe through the second stage. Scuba tank air, as with all properly compressed gasses, is extremely

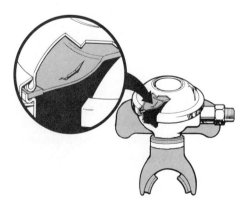

Fig. 1-21 *A split in the demand diaphragm may cause second stage leakage.*

dry and tends to dry out your respiratory tract during a dive. This humidification tends to make breathing scuba tank air more comfortable.

If you intend to do very cold water or ice diving your regulator selection should take into consideration environmental protection so as to not be subject to freezing. Most major regulator manufacturers have a line of environmentally protected regulators suitable for cold water diving.

Maintenance

Careful regulator maintenance is needed to prevent rust and salt corrosion from damaging this piece of equipment. The moving parts inside the regulator are built to close tolerances and do not adapt well to foreign material obstructing air passages. All parts are made of stainless steel, brass, teflon, nylon, rubber, or plastic, which are all corrosion-resistant materials. The only way rust can enter a regulator is from the tank. Salt entering the first stage can do harm and may enter if you do not rinse salt from the first stage thoroughly after a dive, ensuring that water does not enter the regulator itself. When the salt dries, it forms crystals that can build up, cause friction between moving parts, may cause breathing difficulties, and in some cases, may completely stop the flow of air.

Another major cause of leaks in the first stage is faulty or unlubricated "O" rings. This can also cause leaks in the low-pressure hose at the connections, or it could be that the hose needs to be tightened in these areas. Leaks or water in the second stage may stem from a faulty demand diaphragm, as shown in Fig. 1-21, or a deformed diaphragm seat, as in Fig. 1-22. Any leakage from either the first or second stage indicates the need for maintenance by a professional regulator repair technician.

Other problems, such as adjustments or any overhauling of one internal mechanism in either the first or second stage, in addition to the problems just discussed, absolutely require that you take the regulator in for professional service. Regulator repair is beyond the realm of recreational divers. In any event, regulators that are used on a regular basis should be serviced at least once a year and more often if they are used heavily in the ocean. This is vital if your regulator is to function at peak efficiency at all times.

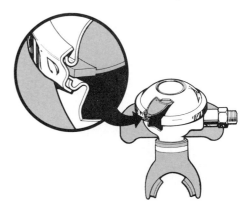

Fig. 1-22 Damage to the second stage regulator housing may result in damage to the seat of the exhaust diaphragm.

The more conscientious you are about caring for your regulator, the less professional maintenance it will need and the less money you will have to spend on this maintenance. Good regulator care actually begins with using it properly under water.

Divers can be quite a spectacle underwater when wearing dive gear, and this is amplified if various hoses are floating at different angles from your body (see Fig. 1-23). This is not only an eyesore and a hindrance to your swimming ability, it can also be hazardous. If not secured to your body, the various hoses coming off the first stage of the regulator (the octopus second stage, submersible pressure gauge or console, power inflator for the BC, and your own primary second stage [when you are snorkeling]), may become entangled in rocks, kelp, and lines. This can damage the hoses and the regulator itself. If you are passing through heavy surf, it is possible for instruments attached to the hoses to fly up and hit you, causing possible injury. Damage to delicate corals may also occur if you are reef diving.

It is very important to secure the octopus second stage to keep it from free-flowing, becoming fouled with sand or mud, or creating confusion in an emergency. Stow the octopus regulator near your chest so you or your buddy has access to it

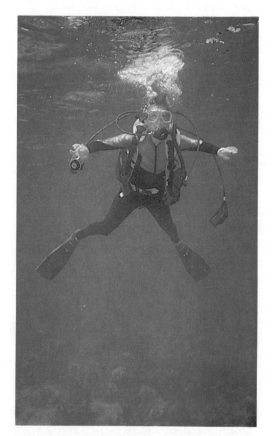

Fig. 1-23 *Poor control of yourself and your equipment poses a threat to you as well as to the environment around you.*

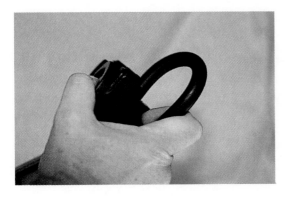

Fig. 1-24 A defective hose will bulge if it is bent at a 45-degree angle.

Fig. 1-25 Stress sleeves or hose protectors help to reduce strain or wear on hoses as they exit the first stage.

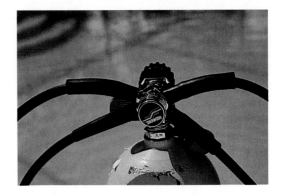

during an out-of-air situation and so you can reach it easily if your primary second stage regulator should malfunction.

Another reason for keeping your hoses under control is to reduce drag on the hoses. This can weaken them in the area where hoses are attached to the first stage. A good way to see if this has happened is to bend the hose at about a 45-degree angle as shown in Fig. 1-24, and if you notice a bulge, change the hose as soon as possible. Otherwise, the hose could rupture, which shuts off the supply of air from the cylinder and fills the hose and regulator with water. You can prevent much of the strain placed on hoses by using commercial stress sleeves, sometimes called *hose protectors* (see Fig. 1-25). If you use hose protectors, periodically check under the protector sleeves for hose damage.

At the end of your dive, you should not leave the regulator on a tank that is standing upright, because this also puts a strain on the hoses. When you remove the regulator from the tank, blow the dust cap dry orally or dry it with a towel. If you use tank air to dry the dust cap, be careful to not blow water into the regulator inlet. When the cap has been thoroughly dried, place it over the high pressure inlet of the first stage and tighten the yoke screw for a good seal. Be sure not to damage the "O" ring or the dust cap itself by tightening the yoke screw too much.

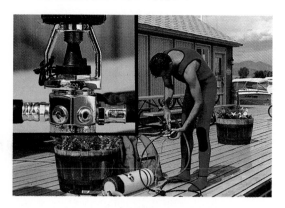

Fig. 1-26 *Proper positioning for the second stage while rinsing after a dive.*

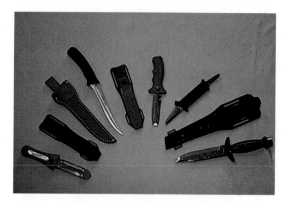

Fig. 1-27 *A wide variety of knives and diving tools are available to the diver.*

A better type of dust cap is plastic with a solid core in the center and an "O" ring on the bottom for a seal. The "O" ring provides a proper seal. Once the dust cap is in place, rinse the first stage with fresh, warm water. Flush the ports for about 2 minutes to dilute any salt and to wash out any sand that may have accumulated inside. Since sand collects even more easily in the large chamber of the second stage, rinse it for about 3 minutes. Hold the exhaust tee at the lowest point and let water flow into the mouthpiece and out the exhaust tee, as shown in Fig. 1-26. Do not push the purge button when you are doing this, as sand and salt crystals may enter the valve and go through the hose into the first stage, causing regulator malfunction. Remember, never let water enter the high pressure inlet of the first stage. If fresh water ever gets into your first stage, blow it out immediately. If salt water gets into the first stage, rinse it out with fresh water then blow it out.

Always lay the regulator down rather than hanging it by the yoke. When the regulator is allowed to hang, the hoses bend slightly and the weight of the second stage breaks down the hose fibers. Also, be careful not to coil the hoses tightly during storage; this can also weaken the hoses. Keep the regulator out of direct sunlight, because too much sunlight can cause rapid deterioration of the rubber. Instead, store it in a dark, cool, dry place.

Using silicone to lubricate your regulator hoses and working metal parts to prevent malfunction has several drawbacks:

1. Although silicone is considered nontoxic, if used in large quantities, it could become toxic at greater than average depths.
2. Silicone can become gummy if sprayed inside the regulator.
3. It may make the edge of the diaphragm slippery and when silicone goes through the rubber pores and into the clamping areas of the diaphragm, it is possible for the diaphragm to become unseated.
4. It may cause rubber, such as the low-pressure diaphragm and the exhale valve, to warp.
5. Sand may cling to areas sprayed with silicone.

Silicone can be effective for smooth regulator function if used properly. Only qualified regulator repair technicians should use silicone when the regulator is undergoing regular maintenance.

KNIFE

The type of knife you own depends primarily on how you intend to use it (Fig. 1-27). Carry the knife where it is easiest to reach. Spots favored by divers include the inner lower leg opposite the strong hand, outer thigh, inner wrist, and the hip. Very small dive knives now available on the market also strap very comfortably to the front shoulder strap of your BC. If the knife is worn on the lower leg around the calf as shown in Fig. 1-28, it will not get caught on objects, such as kelp or fish lines. If you wear the knife on your thigh, attach it either in a knife pocket or by fasteners. This allows for additional comfort and ease of attachment without the restriction and insecurity of the straps. Inner wrist and chest mounts place the knife in an easily accessible position and where it is unlikely to become entangled in line or other objects. All of these knife-mount locations take into consideration not only ease of accessibility but also that the placement will allow limited environmental

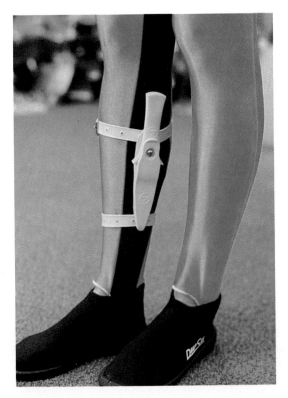

Fig. 1-28 Knives should be worn so as not to be an impediment nor to permit any damage to the environment. (Courtesy of Julie Bauer.)

damage from a protruding object from the diver's body. When your knife becomes dull, do not hone it, rather, sharpen it with a fine file. The serrated edge thus produced will more easily and quickly cut line.

Information Equipment

So many subtle, yet critical things happen to the body under pressure, that it is necessary to monitor physical changes while diving. The increased pressure causes the body to absorb more gasses, and if you stay down longer and dive deeper that gas absorption increases even more. As a result, you must determine how long you are down and how deep you go, while also monitoring your air supply and maintaining awareness of the water temperature.

At this stage in your training, you should be familiar with the equipment that provides underwater orientation and can keep you within safe diving depths. Knowing that your submersible pressure gauge, depth gauge, compass, watch or dive timer, and dive computer are all working properly because of regular maintenance can certainly make your dives much more comfortable and relaxing. You will not have to wonder if you have exceeded your depth limits because you will know your depth gauge is accurately calibrated, and you will be assured your compass is guiding you in the right direction because you have regularly checked it and maintained it as you would any similar instrument.

SUBMERSIBLE PRESSURE GAUGE

There should be no question about why it is important to continuously monitor your air supply. To run out of air underwater not only marks you as a poor diver but is also dangerous. With the rare exception of gauge failure, there is simply no excuse to ever unknowingly run out of air. The only accurate way to monitor your air consumption is with a submersible pressure gauge (SPG). Purchased separately, it is generally available in one quality level and therefore requires little comment. Several SPGs are shown in Fig. 1-29. With the advent of today's modern LCD diving computer-console combinations, tank pressure is simply one of several items of information being presented to the diver (see Fig. 1-30). As with the computer shown, an interesting feature of some computer-console combinations is that they report back to the diver bottom time remaining based upon rate of air consumption with a safe reserve if the air consumption rate would put the diver in greater danger than the maximum bottom time remaining based upon the decompression situation. If you are using a computer and are fortunate enough to have a first stage regulator with two high-pressure ports, you can "back up" your computer by installing a conventional SPG along with the computer.

Maintenance

The most common problems with pressure gauges are leaks, generally caused by dried "O" rings or damage from rough use. Cleaning, replacement, and lubrication at a qualified repair facility will correct these problems. You should also take your gauge in for repair if you notice any moisture under the lens or if you suspect that

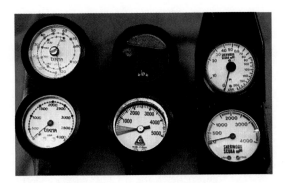 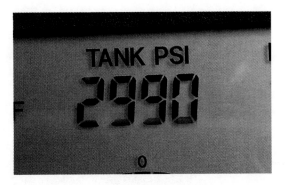

Fig. 1-29 *A representative collection of SPGs. As you can see they are all essentially the same.*

Fig. 1-30 *Like several diving computers on the market, remaining cylinder pressure is simply one of several data items being reported back to the diver constantly.*

salt water and other contaminants have entered the internal mechanism. Qualified personnel can also make sure all connections in the pressure gauge are tight.

If you notice bubbles coming from the high-pressure hose while diving, replace it. This hose should be given the same type of treatment as the low-pressure hoses of your second stage(s). When wearing the SPG on a dive, either attach the hose to some other accessible piece of equipment (your console), or tuck it into a pocket or strap of your BC. This keeps the SPG convenient for checking and prevents it from picking up sand and debris as it drags along the bottom, which might either damage the calibration of the gauge mechanism or mar the lens face. You may want to consider the use of a protective rubber housing for your SPG.

The pressure gauge lens receives the most wear. Scratches, nicks, and cuts can be polished with a fine, mild abrasive to let you see the pressure scale clearly but this corrective action may weaken the lens. Underwater, scratches are not a problem as water fills them in and the gauge becomes clear.

RESERVE SYSTEMS

At one time, it was suggested that reserve systems were alternatives to the pressure gauge. They are not actually viable alternatives as they should be used as a back-up to the pressure gauge. There are two types of reserve systems. The constant reserve is a mechanical lever, called the "J" valve, which operates by spring tension, allowing air to pass through the valve down to a preset level of 300 to 600 psi. When the pressure reaches the preset level, the spring moves a pin into the air passage and greatly restricts the air supply. At that point, the reserve spring can be mechanically bypassed to provide an additional 300 to 600 psi of air. One of the problems of using the system alone is that 300 to 600 psi, under certain diving circumstances, may not be sufficient to allow a proper, safe ascent. Another type of reserve is the audible reserve, which activates on low air pressure. It too serves to back up the SPG. Since SPGs at a minimum are standard equipment for recre-

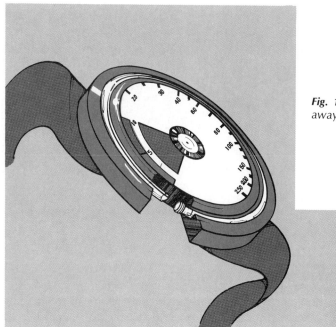

Fig. 1-31 The capillary depth gauge and a cut-away of the depth measuring mechanism.

ational diving, reserve systems are a redundancy. However, since equipment failures and leaks do occur, even in situations where equipment is well cared for, reserve systems simply serve as a back-up and should be properly maintained if you have them.

DEPTH GAUGE

The depth gauge is a device that tells you how deep you are. Below 30 feet, it becomes increasingly important to accurately measure your depth. On ascent, it becomes very important to accurately monitor depths in the shallower waters of 30 feet or less. This information is important in avoiding problems with decompression and in estimating your rate of air consumption, which, of course, varies with depth. Depth gauges can become inaccurate with normal use and should be tested periodically. There are four kinds of depth gauge: capillary, bourdon tube, diaphragm, and electronic.

The capillary gauge is perhaps the simplest since it has no moving parts and operates on the basic principle of Boyle's law (see Fig. 1-31). It has an air-filled tube sealed at one end. The air inside the tube compresses as water pressure increases. When you descend to 33 feet, the ambient pressure doubles and the volume is halved, as shown in Fig. 1-32. This natural law makes it possible to accurately measure depth down to approximately 60 feet. Beyond 60 feet, the percentage of pres-

Fig. 1-32 In reaction to Boyle's law, the volume of air in the capillary tube is compressed to one-half of its volume at 33 feet.

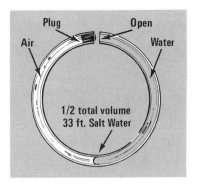

sure change is less and the graduations on the capillary gauge are closer together, which makes the gauge much more difficult to read.

Both the open and closed bourdon tube depth gauges, as shown in Figs. 1-33 and 1-34, work on the same principle. Ambient pressure is transmitted to the mechanism of the gauge, called the **C** spring, which is a hollow spring in the shape of a **C**. This transfer of pressure straightens the spring. This motion, in turn, is transferred to the dial mechanism. The difference between the open and closed bourdon tube is that water passes through the opening in the side of the open bourdon tube gauge to straighten the spring. In the closed bourdon tube depth gauge, surrounding pressure from all directions is transmitted from outside to the liquid surrounding the inner mechanism. Pressure is then transmitted to the **C** spring and on to the dial. Because it is sealed from the water, the closed bourdon tube gauge is

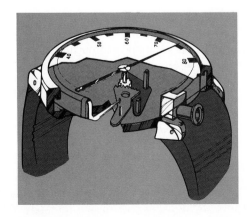

Fig. 1-33 Cut-away view of the open bourdon tube depth gauge.

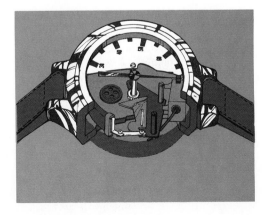

Fig. 1-34 Cut-away view of the closed bourdon tube depth gauge.

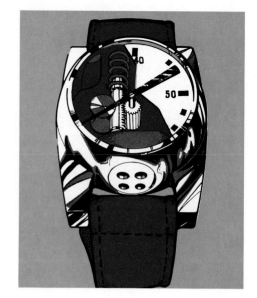

Fig. 1-35 Cut-away view of the diaphragm depth gauge.

much more dependable, less subject to corrosion, and much more accurate than the capillary or open bourdon tube gauges. It is also more durable because the oil cushions the gears inside, which protects the calibration should the gauge be dropped.

The diaphragm depth gauge, as shown in Fig. 1-35, has a diaphragm stretched over an opening in the air filled housing. The diaphragm moves as pressure increases, which starts a chain reaction in the mechanism between the diaphragm and the needle on the face of the gauge. The needle then records the depth on the scale. Most diaphragm gauges have an accuracy of between 2% and 5%.

Closely related to the diaphragm depth gauge insofar as the way it responds to the ambient environment is the most accurate type of gauge—the electronic depth gauge. A sensor, similar to the diaphragm depth gauge's diaphragm, reacts to the ambient pressure. This pressure is evaluated by an electronic sensor that converts this "analog" information to the "digital" depth information read on the face of the gauge.

Some bourdon tube and diaphragm gauges are equipped with a separate needle that registers the maximum depth of the dive. Electronic gauges use a small computer memory element to record this information and report it back, digitally, to the diver. Most electronic depth gauges also store and report back to the diver the bottom time and surface interval time between dives.

Maintenance

Maintenance for depth gauges primarily involves a thorough rinsing to prevent corrosion, but all three types of gauge require slightly different rinsing methods. For the capillary gauge, you must first carefully remove the gauge tube and connection insert, flush these with fresh water, and push a pipe cleaner through the tube. When you reassemble the device, make sure the insert that holds the two ends of the tube faces the left end of the tube and has the notched side up. If the tube is not replaced properly, the gauge will register backward.

Since the open bourdon tube depth gauge has a very small opening in the case, it is subject to corrosion and plugging from impurities, and you need sufficient water pressure to clean it. Dental water jet devices do a good job. Let the gauge register to 30 feet several times while you rinse it. You can also submerge the pressure gauge in water while you are rinsing the port. Another method for eliminating corrosion is to immerse the gauge in white vinegar for a short time, rinse it thoroughly with clear water, and lubricate it with a light lubricant, such as silicone. Do not leave your depth gauge in the vinegar too long, because it is a mild acid that could cause damage. It is only necessary to rinse the exteriors of both oil-filled bourdon tube, diaphragm, and electronic depth gauges with water because they have no open ports. Extremes in heat and cold can affect all gauges, so protect depth gauges from temperature extremes.

The greatest wear comes from abrasion and scuffing of the lens cover. Polishing with a mild abrasive removes scuffs to a large extent. You should have the depth gauge regularly checked for accurate calibration but, if you discover a discrepancy in accuracy or any kind of internal damage at any time, take the depth gauge in for professional repair.

COMPASS

The underwater compass comes in three basic models: the small watchband compass that fits on the band of the watch or depth gauge, the top-reading wrist compass, and the side-reading wrist compass. The wrist models generally fit into a console or they can be used individually. The higher quality wrist models are much more desirable for underwater navigation. Watchband compasses are generally for appearance and give only general directional indications. The other compass styles allow more precise navigation.

Maintenance

Basic compass maintenance includes loose or sticky components or damage to the compass card. In all cases, keep the exterior clean and well-lubricated with silicone grease, as opposed to silicone spray. You should also transport the compass carefully. The compass is a delicate instrument and will not stand up to heavy abuse. Damage to the compass often is not repairable and calls for replacement.

CONSOLE

One answer to the profusion of gauges that may hang from a diver's body is the instrument panel, also called a console (see Fig. 1-36). This device encloses the submersible pressure gauge, depth gauge, compass, and sometimes the dive computer in one unit mounted on the pressure gauge hose. An option to this is to attach the depth gauge on the back of the SPG. There are units made especially for

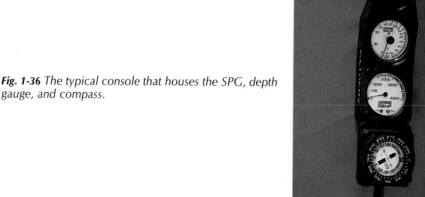

Fig. 1-36 *The typical console that houses the SPG, depth gauge, and compass.*

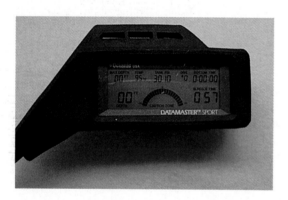

Fig. 1-37 *This single device replaces all of the instruments found on a console except the compass, which can be mounted on the back of this unit.*

this purpose. The other gauges are worn separately on the wrist or in pockets. Because the metal in other gauges may affect the magnetism of the compass, it works more accurately when you wear it separately from the other gauges. When mounting your compass, consider all ferrous metals (iron or steel) that may be used in tanks or other metal parts that may affect your compass readings. Some recent innovations in diving equipment include single units that include the dive computer and all gauges in one single unit as shown in Fig. 1-37.

Whether you use a console, separate pressure gauge, or all-inclusive computer, the assembly should be secured near the front of the BC, with the hose routed under the left arm to permit easy scanning of the gauges. The gauge, console, or computer are mounted on the lower left margin of the BC or on the left thigh. This position keeps the console from becoming entangled.

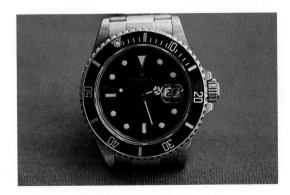

Fig. 1-38 *The indicator may be set at the end of the time for your dive plan.*

Fig. 1-39 *The indicator may be set at the time you initiate your descent and you will note bottom time on the bezel at the time of your ascent.*

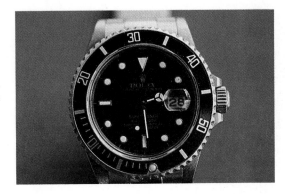

DIVE WATCH

If your diving watch is pressure-proof well beyond whatever depth you intend to dive, it should cause you no problems. The better quality dive watches have such features as mineral crystals, a higher-quality inner mechanism, and significantly greater durability than other watches. They can withstand more abuse and, of course, have increased accuracy.

The most critical part of the analog (with "hands" not digits) dive watch is the bezel. You can use it two ways: either set the indicator at the end of amount of time you wish to be down, as shown in Fig. 1-38, or set the indicator at the time you went down and take note of the bottom time on the bezel at the time of your ascent, as shown in Fig. 1-39.

Dive timers or digital dive watches may be somewhat easier to read underwater. Some digital watches also feature a digital display that automatically tracks bottom time by using pressure to turn off and on (Fig. 1-40). The best watch band to use on diving watches is one that passes through both retaining pins. Bands that attach separately to each side of the watch may be lost if one retaining pin falls out during a dive.

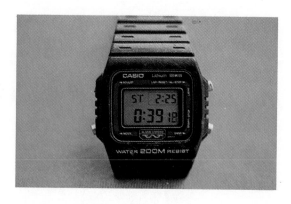

Fig. 1-40 *Digital watches or bottom timers may be easier to read underwater and some have added features for tracking bottom time.*

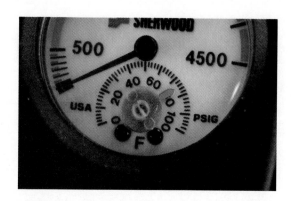

Fig. 1-41 *Waterproof and pressure-proof thermometer.*

THERMOMETER

To prevent hypothermia and to let you know what degree of diving protection to use, it is important that you monitor ambient water temperatures. A simple thermometer, as shown in Fig. 1-41, is all that is required and is more than accurate enough to clearly indicate ambient temperature both above and below the water.

COMPUTERS

In the *Open Water Sport Diver Manual* diving computers were briefly discussed and a list of safety rules were given. This manual teaches the diver a little more about the computers and gives an expanded explanation of the reasoning behind the safety rules.

As an experienced diver, you are already aware of the dangers of excess nitrogen saturation in the body and Chapter 10 will explore in greater depth the problems associated with decompression sickness. Dive computers calculate the theoretical uptake and elimination of nitrogen for a diver throughout diving activities.

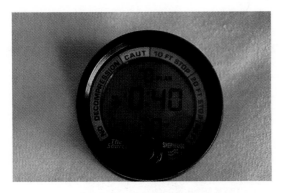 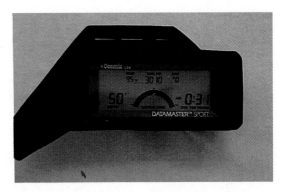

Figs. 1-42 and 1-43 *Computers can be more complex and offer a wide array of features in addition to the decompression computer.*

There is no need for calculations and the dive computer automatically keeps track of time and depth for the diver. There is a wide variety of computers now available in the marketplace offering a wide array of features and benefits, including dive profile data, air consumption, and temperature (Figs. 1-42 and 1-43). The primary benefit of all dive computers, however, is their ability to perform multilevel dive calculations.

Computers offer some advantages over dive tables. The principal feature of a dive computer is that it is a dynamic dive monitor, actually making the dive with the diver. The dive computer is continually calculating the diver's decompression status with regard to dive time, depth, and theoretical nitrogen in-gassing and outgassing. By contrast, dive tables are a static device that help to calculate the same information based solely on the maximum depth attained and the length of time underwater.

The difference between dive computers and dive tables becomes readily apparent during multilevel dives. Most divers rarely go to a single depth and actually stay there for the entire dive. Diving in a variety of depth segments during the course of a single dive is known as multilevel diving.

A multilevel diver using dive tables is penalized by having to use the maximum depth attained for all dive calculations. In reality, the diver may have spent only a small portion of the dive at the maximum depth while the majority of the dive may have been spent at shallower depths where the nitrogen uptake within the body or in-gassing will have been slower. The table diver calculates as if the entire dive is performed at the maximum depth, thus assuming a maximum level of nitrogen absorption or in-gassing. In contrast, a dive computer is constantly calculating during all depth segments of the dive and gives credit for the shallower portions of the dive where in-gassing is slower or where a diver may even be out-gassing. The net result is that a diver using a set of dive tables for the calculation of decompression status generally will be allowed much less time underwater than if the diver had been using a dive computer that had been continuously calculating theoretical nitrogen status based on actual depth and time spent at that depth.

A final benefit of the dive computers is that they require no dive table calculations. This eliminates the potential for diver error placing a diver in jeopardy.

It is important to remember that dive computers are merely electronic devices that account for the theoretical absorption and elimination of nitrogen within a diver's body based upon a series of mathematical models. Computers do not monitor stress, exercise level, or fitness. In other words, dive computers are simply accounting tools that help a diver make decisions in order to prevent decompression sickness. It cannot be overemphasized that these devices are not calculating actual nitrogen level within a diver's body. Dive computers must be used wisely as a guide in making decisions to avoid decompression sickness.

Safe Utilization of Computers

In order to help a diver use a dive computer wisely and consequently reduce the risk of decompression sickness, a series of guidelines are given. Using these dive guidelines and a dive computer wisely can greatly reduce the risk of injury due to decompression sickness.

One of the first and most important procedures that a diver can follow is to be thoroughly familiar with the operation of the particular computer in use. There are a variety of different dive computers available and each one has its own special parameters of operation and usage limitations. The importance of being properly trained in the operation of the dive computer cannot be overemphasized. Many dive computer manufacturers have developed educational videos and user workbooks to accompany their owner manuals. Additional training may be obtained by enrolling in a dive computer specialty course offered through your instructor or dive store.

After becoming thoroughly familiar with the operation and limitations of the computer, there are rules that should be followed to enhance diver safety and reduce the risk of decompression sickness. Many of these concepts are identical to the concepts learned for using the dive tables. This makes sense since the dive computer is performing the same theoretical nitrogen accounting task as the dive tables, but in a different manner. These diving safety guidelines are as follows:

1. Each diver should use his or her own dive computer. More specifically, each diver should maintain responsibility for his or her own decompression status whether using a dive computer or dive table. Dive computers constantly make calculations with respect to depth, time, and decompression status during a dive. Each diver's profile may be slightly different and, as a consequence, the decompression status is calculated specifically to that dive profile.

2. Divers should dive conservatively with respect to the no-decompression limits. This is an excellent idea whether using a dive computer or dive table. Be aware that some dive computers are more conservative than others with respect to no-decompression limits. Remember that a dive computer is essentially an electronic monitor that accounts for theoretical nitrogen uptake and

release based on a mathematical model. Therefore, use it as a tool and do not push its limits as many people have different susceptibilities to decompression sickness.

3. Diving conservatively while using a dive computer includes performing only no-decompression diving. All of the dive computers available have the capability to perform decompression calculations for a diver. A decompression stop is a pause or stop during the ascent at a specified depth for a specified time period to allow for the gradual elimination of nitrogen. In reality, to make a decompression stop using a dive computer appears to be simple. It is important to realize that a diver in a decompression mode has lost the ability to ascend directly to the surface. As a consequence, any situation that might require a direct ascent to the surface could be a potential problem causing decompression sickness. A primary consideration is whether or not the diver has a sufficient air supply to make any required decompression stops. Additionally, any emergencies that would require a direct ascent to the surface, such as running out of air, rupturing an air hose, or even having a buddy that runs out of air, could result in disaster since a diver in a decompression mode should not ascend directly to the surface. Decompression diving is beyond the realm of recreational diving because of the risks and should not be undertaken.

4. All ascents should be slow so as to not exceed the computer specified ascent rates. All of the dive computers currently available have some form of ascent rate monitor. Most of these monitors specify slower ascent rates than the U.S. Navy dive table ascent rate of 60 feet per minute. Slower ascent rates have also been shown to help prevent the formation of nitrogen bubbles in divers. All divers should monitor their computer during the ascent, being careful not to exceed the computer specified ascent rate, which will greatly reduce the risk of decompression sickness.

5. In addition to slow ascents from depth, it has been demonstrated that safety stops are beneficial in the prevention of decompression sickness. Diving conservatively should include a safety stop on every dive at approximately 15 feet for 3 to 5 minutes.

6. In a series of repetitive dives, the deepest dive should be made first. Making the deepest dive first maximizes bottom time and decreases the risk of decompression sickness. Multilevel dives should be initiated with the deepest segment of the dive first and subsequent portions of the dive should be made in progressively shallower water. Repetitive dives to depths in excess of 100 feet should be avoided.

7. As was previously stated, dive computers constantly calculate the theoretical levels of nitrogen within a diver's body during a dive. In addition, they also calculate the theoretical rate of release or out-gassing of nitrogen during a surface interval. Accordingly, a dive computer should never be turned off between dives or before it has calculated complete out-gassing. This is another reason why dive computers should not be shared since they account for the theoretical uptake and release of an individual diver throughout the entire day's diving activity including surface intervals between dives.

8. Dive computers are dependable and rarely fail. However, it is still a good idea to be familiar with the proper procedures in the event of a computer failure. There are two areas of possible failure. The dive computer could fail during a dive or it might fail during a surface interval between dives.

a. The procedure if the computer stops functioning during a dive is relatively simple. The diver should ascend to the surface, going as slowly as possible and making a safety stop at approximately 15 feet for 3 to 5 minutes. Additionally, if the computer were to stop functioning during a decompression mode, the diver would have no way of monitoring the proper decompression stop. This is another reason why decompression diving should be avoided.

b. The procedure for diving when a computer fails between dives is also straightforward. A computer failure during a surface interval actually leaves a diver with three alternatives. The first alternative is to make a single repetitive dive using the adjusted no-decompression limit or dive time remaining limit given by the computer during its surface interval scrolling mode before the failure. Alternatively, repetitive dives could be made to depths of less than 30 feet. The third alternative is to end the day's diving activities. An additional consideration is what to do the next day if the computer is either repaired or another unit is obtained. Diving with a computer the next day may present a problem since a full day of diving the previous day may have left the body with residual nitrogen. It has been recommended that there should be no diving within 24 hours before using a new computer or a computer that has been turned off.

9. Many dive computers feature flying after diving indicators that tell a diver when it is safe to fly. Most of these indicators will allow a diver to fly within a short period of time following a day's diving activities. Many authorities are currently recommending that recreational divers wait 12 to 24 hours after diving before flying. Waiting this additional period of time certainly adds an additional margin of safety.

As a final note, dive computers have given divers the freedom of multilevel diving. This freedom has allowed divers to spend more time exploring and enjoying the underwater world. It is important to remember that neither the dive tables nor a dive computer can absolutely ensure that a diver will not get decompression sickness. These devices are based upon mathematical models that have been supported by experimentation and research. Remember to use them properly, following the manufacturer's directions and the dive guidelines recommended here. Using these devices properly and conservatively will greatly decrease the likelihood of injury.

General Equipment Care

You should always rinse your equipment after every dive with clean, fresh, and, preferably, lukewarm water. Since excessive heat can harm most equipment, keep it out of the sun as much as possible and store all pieces at a constant temperature away from polluted areas. If you need to store your gear for a long time, seal each piece individually in chemically stable plastic bags after ensuring everything is completely dry. When silicone and black rubber are stored together in one container, such as a dive bag, the silicone absorbs rubber particles, which causes it to yellow. To prevent staining, seal silicone and black rubber equipment in separate plastic bags or follow the manufacturer's recommendations.

Remember to take both your tank and regulator in for an annual inspection, and more frequently if you detect any damage or breathing resistance. This tip is not limited to the tank and regulator alone. Anything other than the simplest problems normally requires you to take the equipment to a professional repair person for proper maintenance. If you have difficulty with equipment modifications, such as arranging your fin straps, do not be timid; ask for help from your buddy, other divers, your instructor, or the dive store where you purchased the equipment. Most divers have had the same difficulties at one time or another, and all divers should know that the more that can be done to ensure safety on a dive, the better.

2
Specialized Equipment

OBJECTIVES

At the conclusion of this chapter, you should be able to:

1. Explain how the body generates warmth when heat is lost to the water surrounding the diver.
2. Describe the primary consideration in handling a diver who experiences hypothermia.
3. Tell what must be done before giving an injured person fluids by mouth.
4. Name the single most important feature in wet suit selection.
5. State what percentage of heat is lost from the body via heat emanating from the head.
6. Tell at what locations you will find the majority of wet suit leaks.
7. Tell how to signal "stop," "ok," "surface," and "come to me quickly" using a buddy-line.
8. Show how to signal "ok" using a light.
9. Describe the major disadvantage of surface-supplied air sources.
10. Explain the safety standard that should be used when one person in a dive party is using a diver propulsion vehicle.

KEY TERMS

Hypothermia	Pilomotor reflex	Shivering
Manual alphabet	Surface-supplied air	Diver propulsion vehicles

The first level of the learning process is familiarity. At this stage, you may know that your body gets cold underwater and needs protection. You may even know how to protect your body, but there may be a lack of real understanding about why the equipment is so important and exactly how the equipment protects you from the cold.

The goal is to progress to the next level of learning—understanding. This chapter discusses many of the same areas of equipment that have been discussed before, but it presents a new dimension at a level of understanding to help you make well-informed decisions about diving equipment based on something more than familiarity.

Hypothermia

Hypothermia is defined as below-normal body temperature. The word is derived from two Greek words: "hypo" meaning low, and "therme" meaning heat, or low heat. In contrast, hyperthermia is excessive heat. The human body is designed to function at 98.6° F (37° C). Your core stays fairly close to this temperature, even when you "feel" cold. A drop in your core temperature of only a few degrees can cause severe problems. If the temperature drop is not stopped, a series of events begins to occur that can be very serious and even life threatening. Since water draws heat from the body at a rate 25 times greater than air, hypothermia is potentially more serious in water than in air.

SYMPTOMS

Symptoms vary with different levels of hypothermia from mild to severe. Also, the responses of individuals vary with their degree of adaptation to the cold, so the symptoms discussed below may vary from person to person. The first obvious signs that you are getting cold are "goose bumps" on the skin, medically known as a pilomotor reflex, where the hairs on the skin surface stand out and slight shivering may begin. This condition is not serious but should alert a diver that the body is attempting to compensate for what the temperature regulatory system of the body senses to be a threat to a stable core temperature. At this point the core temperature is stable or may have only dropped slightly, and only the extremities are usually affected. If the cold continues, the body will begin to undergo more significant changes. One of the initial defenses of the body is that of the blood vessels on the body's surface tissues constricting to reroute or shunt blood to the core of the body in an effort to maintain core temperature and keep adequate blood flowing to the vital organs.

If immersion in cold water is sudden and involves facial exposure, the diver may experience an additional response to the immersion in addition to shunting. This type of reaction is known as a *vasovagal response:* the heart beat may slow dramatically and suddenly. Although not a response to hypothermia but instead a reaction to cold water contact on certain nerve groups, this is the body's attempt to conserve oxygen and is a part of a number of natural events within the body aimed at survival, and accounting for some remarkable survivals after immersion in cold water.

The changes reflecting hypothermia take place gradually and not in a precise step-wise fashion. The following information, however, is a reflection of the norms relative to changes occurring during hypothermia.

As the core temperature of the body drops further, the symptoms of hypothermia become more pronounced (Table 2-1). In an attempt to replace lost heat, shivering becomes vigorous, body-wide, and continuous. Breathing may become rapid, and hyperventilation may start. As the core temperature reaches 95° F (35° C) the diver may become confused and disoriented, and weakness and loss of coordination may become so pronounced that the diver may not be able to perform necessary tasks.

Table 2-1
Levels of Hypothermia

Temperature		Condition
°F	°C	
99.6	37.6	Normal rectal temperature
98.6	37	Normal oral temperature
96.8	36	Increased metabolic rate
95.0	35	Shivering
93.2	34	Amnesia, difficult speech
91.4	33	Severe hypothermia
90.0	32.2	Shivering stops
89.6	32	Pupils dilated; altered level of consciousness
87.8	31	Blood pressure difficult to obtain
86	30	Progressive loss of consciousness, increased muscle rigidity
85.2	29	Slower pulse and respiration
82.4	28	Cardiac problems develop
80.6	27	Voluntary motion lost along with pupillary light reflexes; the patient may appear dead
78.8	26	Patient seldom conscious

From Judd RL, Ponsell DD: *Mosby's first responder,* ed 2, St Louis, 1988, Mosby–Year Book, p 324.

If the core temperature is further reduced to 90° F (32° C), the diver becomes sleepy and lethargic and experiences muscle rigidity, his or her breathing becomes shallow, and he or she may lose consciousness. By the time this temperature is reached, shivering will have stopped and the body will have lost its ability to rewarm itself.

If the temperature continues to drop, without aggressive medical intervention, cardiac rhythm disturbances and death will soon follow.

Other factors may contribute to hypothermia or make the symptoms worse. Fatigue, nitrogen narcosis, anxiety, and residual alcohol can compound the body's response to reduced temperatures. When diving in waters 40° F or colder, sudden immersion may be fatal, even before the central core temperature begins to drop. Finally, when doing repetitive dives in a cold environment, heat loss may continue and reach a dangerous level if the diver does not rewarm between dives.

Treatment and Prevention

A major consideration in the treatment of a diver with hypothermia is that the victim should be handled as gently as possible. Abrupt or rough handling of the hypothermic diver may initiate a lethal heart rhythm, ventricular fibrillation.

If you suspect a diver to be hypothermic, the primary consideration should be the stabilization of body temperature and the prevention of further heat loss. If the diver is still in the water, get him or her out. Water drains body heat 25 times faster than air, so the diver must be quickly taken from the water. All wet or frozen clothing or dive gear should be removed, and the victim should be wrapped in warm blankets. Those areas of the body that should be especially protected from heat loss are the head, neck, and trunk. If the diver is still conscious and oriented, begin rewarming by moving the diver into a heated environment and administering warm fluids by mouth. You should recognize, though, that ingestion of warmed fluids will only slightly influence a hypothermic condition and is virtually of no value in the severely hypothermic diver regardless of the diver's ability to tolerate oral fluids. Before giving injured individuals any fluids by mouth, you must be sure they are conscious and alert, can swallow, and are not shivering so uncontrollably that they might choke on the liquid being swallowed. Do not give hypothermic individuals either coffee or alcohol. Alcohol contributes significantly to the rate and amount of body heat lost, whereas the caffeine stimulant in coffee may exacerbate cardiac side-effects.

If the diver is unconscious, the following steps should be taken:

1. If the diver is not breathing, begin mouth-to-mask or mouth-to-mouth ventilation as quickly as possible.
2. If you can detect a pulse, *DO NOT* begin cardiopulmonary resuscitation (CPR). If you cannot feel a pulse at the carotid artery, begin CPR.
3. Be gentle in handling the victim. Avoid any unnecessary handling and manipulation of the neck and limbs.
4. Do not attempt to initiate any measures to rewarm the victim. The methods to do so and means employed should be left to the medical personnel to whom you will transfer the victim. Rapid rewarming of the victim in the wrong fashion is potentially fatal.
5. The most important intervention is to maintain the victim's body temperature and prevent any further heat loss by removing any wet garments or equipment and wrapping the victim in dry blankets.
6. Attempt to stabilize any injuries other than the hypothermia provided you know how to do so.
7. Transport the victim to a medical care facility as rapidly as possible without endangering either the victim or yourself.

The possibility of hypothermia should be taken very seriously and you should take measures to avoid it at all times. Most people will begin to shiver after a loss of 1° to 1.5° C of core temperature. If you begin to shiver violently, get out of the water. Even if you dive in a warm water environment, you are still susceptible to a significant loss of body heat. A water temperature of 80° F (26° C) may feel warm at first, but the body temperature can be lowered significantly—to the point at which serious results can occur. Because of this, you should wear protection that is appropriate for the type of diving you expect to be doing.

DIVE SKINS

Ultra-thin Lycra material has been used to provide protection for divers who dive in warm water; divers who desire a minimal thermal protection and protection from

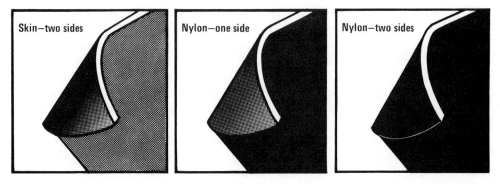

Fig. 2-1 *A guide to wet suit thickness appropriate for ambient diving temperatures expected.*

abrasion. *Skins,* as they have become known, are sometimes worn under wet suits and dry suits. Most skins are made from a Lycra material that may or may not be impregnated with neoprene for added warmth.

WET SUIT PROTECTION

Neoprene is available in several thicknesses. Thicker neoprene, naturally, provides more insulation. After a point, however, there is a trade-off between the increased warmth and the increased effort required to move inside the stiffer, heavier material. Fig. 2-1 gives recommended wet suit thicknesses relative to water temperature where diving activities take place. Before selecting the type of suit you need, you should also consider your activity level. If you are quite active, a slightly lighter than average suit may be appropriate. A thinner suit gives you more flexibility and less resistance. On the other hand, if you are not very active underwater, you should wear a thicker wet suit because it increases insulation, and the resistance and stiffness of the material may not be a significant factor.

Wet suits are constructed three different ways. You can choose from suits that are unlined (skin–two side), lined with nylon on one side only (nylon–one side), or lined with nylon on both sides (nylon–two side). Most modern suits have nylon or Lycra on both sides. Lycra and nylon are most generally used for lining; however, manufacturers have been testing many fabrics to determine their warmth, comfort, and durability. Nylon and Lycra have the added benefit of allowing for a vast array of color combinations, a welcome alternative to the once drab diving attire.

There are advantages and disadvantages of having material adhered to the neoprene. The skin–two side type of suit has the most flexibility. It can be cut tighter to the body, which decreases the circulation of water under the suit and keeps you warmer than a suit with nylon bonded to one or both sides. The disadvantages are that the neoprene alone is not very strong and the seams are bonded with glue, which does not hold the seams together adequately. Bare neoprene also tears quite easily, and the nature of the material makes it difficult to put on and take off.

Having nylon on one side of the neoprene is better for wear and durability because the seams can be sewn on one side, which gives it more strength. Having nylon on the inside makes it easier to don and doff the suit; however, it still permits snagging and tearing on the outside. If the suit is lined only on the outside, the tearing and snagging problem is reduced, but the problem of getting into and out of the suit still remains.

Suits with material on two sides eliminate most of the problems. Many suits today are lined with "plush" material for ease of donning and comfort, are more durable, do not snag, and have stronger seams than the other two types of wet suit. The disadvantages of having nylon on two sides are added stiffness, which increases somewhat with age, and reduced flexibility. However, with the improvements in fabric technology and the introduction of newer wet suit fabrics, these problems are diminishing significantly. Notably, Lycra-lined suits provide for easier donning and have all the advantages of nylon.

WET SUIT SELECTION

The critical areas of protection are the groin, trunk, small of the back, under the arms, neck, and, most significantly, the head. Two things determine how much protection a wet suit provides: general fit, and the amount of material or insulation in the critical areas mentioned.

Excellent fit is the most important feature of a wet suit. A ³⁄₁₆-inch wet suit that fits well is warmer than one that is thicker and heavier but does not fit as well. For most divers, a custom-made suit is best. For a suit to fit correctly, it should feel like a second skin—snug everywhere and not tight enough to restrict motion, but certainly tight enough to avoid circulation of water. A wet suit is warmer if the amount of water circulation is limited. If your diving is going to be limited to relatively warm waters, the off-the-rack wet suit will probably be adequate, or, if you know someone skilled in sewing and repair of wet suits, you can select a stock wet suit that fits pretty well and then have it modified to the perfect fit. Fig. 2-2 is an example of one of the attractive wet suits that can be purchased in standard sizes.

The hood and boots should be snug but not too tight. It is important that the hood opening around the face be small enough to allow a proper seal with the mask as shown in Fig. 2-3. In colder water diving, the hood is perhaps the most significant of all the protective items a diver may wear, since approximately 40% of all heat loss emanates from the head. To fit correctly, wet suit gloves should be tight enough to prevent water circulation but loose enough not to cause cramping.

For diving in warmer waters, above 80° F, the trunk, groin, and underarms are the areas typically protected. Although a wet suit vest might be all that is necessary for this protection, the ideal wet suit for this type of diving would be the shorty (Fig. 2-4), as this type of suit protects the vulnerable areas mentioned. If a diver is particularly susceptible to the cold (for example, a diver with Raynaud's disease), then a hood is probably a necessary piece of diving wear regardless of the environment.

For waters with temperatures in the 80s in which the diver feels comfortable, the very light full-suit or Lycra dive skins probably provide all that is necessary for most divers. However, it should be remembered that comfort is paramount when it comes to warmth and cold. The degree of protection required to keep you comfort-

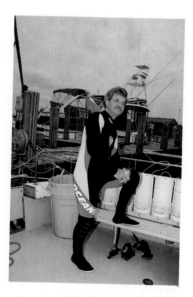

Fig. 2-2 A properly fitting wet suit suitable for anticipated diving conditions.

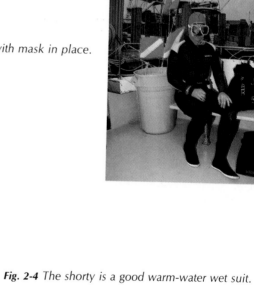

Fig. 2-3 Properly fitted hood with mask in place.

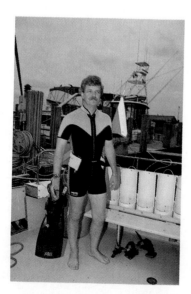

Fig. 2-4 The shorty is a good warm-water wet suit.

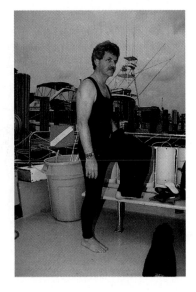

Fig. *2-5 The Farmer John provides a double layer of wet suit material around the trunk.*

able is a decision that can be made only by one person—*you*. Just because some of your diving companions can get by with dive skins and you need a full wet suit for the same degree of comfort, do not let them intimidate you into hypothermia. Wear whatever degree of protection it takes to keep you warm and comfortable. You will notice that your need for protection may tend to vary with adaptation— the more used to certain diving temperatures that you and your body become, the less your need for protective garments.

For waters between 72° F (22° C) and 80° F (27° C) the areas of the body that need protection are essentially the same as for warmer waters. However, if you will be exposed to these water temperatures you should consider the addition of a diving hood. The best suits for this purpose are the one-piece jumpsuit, as shown in Fig. 2-2, or the Farmer John suit shown in Fig. 2-5, a suit that provides a double layer of wet suit protection around the trunk. An alternative, to add a margin of warmth to the trunk, would be to wear a diving vest under the wet suit.

When you dive in cold water, between 50° F (10° C) and 70° F (21° C), you need to protect your body as thoroughly as possible. The body cools very rapidly and requires a full suit along with hood, boots, and gloves in the coldest ranges of this temperature range. It becomes critical to protect the head, neck, hands, and feet. An adequate suit for this type of water is a jumpsuit with a vest or a standard two-piece suit with a vest, including hood, boots, and gloves. You can use other options as long as the protection of the body is complete. One other option is wearing one of the neoprene-impregnated Lycra dive skins as an undergarment with the wet suit.

For temperatures below 50° F (10° C) some divers use multilayered garments under full wet suit protection with hood, boots, and gloves, but these temperatures are more appropriate for the dry suit, which will be discussed later in this chapter. If you expect to do a great deal of diving in these colder temperature waters, the dry suit is your answer to warmth and comfort.

MAINTENANCE

Problems with wet suits occur most often at the seams. Nylon—one side suits have seams sewn on at least one side. If the suit is a nylon—two side, as are most suits sold today, the seams are sewn on both sides. This double stitching greatly reduces the chances of seam separation. Some manufacturers also place tape on the seam lines. It is good to seal the loose ends of each seam with wet suit cement. Tears are also easily repaired with wet suit cement. The correct way to apply the cement is to spread one light but thorough coat on both surfaces and allow both coats to dry until no longer tacky; then, apply a second coat on both surfaces and allow these coats to dry until they are not too tacky. Finally, join the surfaces and press them together to form a proper seal.

Wet suits receive the most wear at the knees, elbows, and seat. This can be slowed or eliminated by adding pads to these areas. This is done quite simply by cutting additional material and cementing the cut pieces to the wet suit using wet suit cement in the same manner as described for repair of tears. Since photographers and beach divers are on their knees and elbows frequently, they find padding in these areas to be most useful in adding to the life of their wet suits. Gloves tend to wear guite easily and there is little that can be done to prevent this. Plan to replace gloves rather frequently. However, dipping glove fingertips in tool dip will prolong glove life-expectancy.

There are several other wet suit modifications you might consider. One is to add a spine pad. It is designed to keep colder water from flowing down your back by filling in the indentation along your spine. Also, a pocket may be glued to the thigh of your wet suit to hold a knife or other tools. The pocket keeps the knife from moving around your leg or becoming entangled. Another handy addition is a pouch attached to the thigh of the wet suit pants to carry other tools and accessories. When adding any pouches or pockets to the wet suit, you should always be aware of the possible need for emergency removal of gear (for example, weight belt) and make certain that the pouches or pockets will never interfere with these procedures.

The metal swivel fasteners or twist locks on the wet suit jacket's beavertail are prone to corrosion and breakage. Some manufacturers use velcro exclusively today for this closure, and you may wish to replace fasteners with velcro. Otherwise, thoroughly rinse the metal locks after each dive. Zippers, as well as locks, should be lubricated with silicone. If you do not have silicone, use stick lubricant, soap, beeswax, or candle wax to keep them from jamming.

DRY SUIT PROTECTION

Dry suits provide complete thermal protection from the water. As the name implies, they keep you dry. Undergarments can be worn with the suit to help insulate you from the cold, as shown in Fig. 2-6. Dry suits can be constructed of closed-cell or crushed neoprene, fabric, rubber, or laminates. When selecting a dry suit, you should consider the material's durability, resistance to punctures, and ease of repair, among other factors. The more flexible the suit material, the more comfortable it will be. The neck and wrist seals are usually made out of flexible latex or neoprene. Latex seals are more flexible and easier to put on than neoprene, although their service life is shorter. The seals should be firm enough to keep water

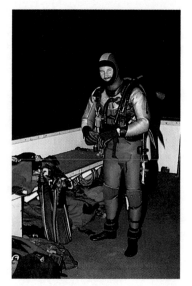

Fig. 2-6 *The typical dry suit used in sport diving. (Courtesy of Matt McDermott.)*

out, yet soft enough to allow normal blood circulation. Talcum powder or warm soapy water makes it easier for you to slip your head and hands through the seals. The zipper location is important for donning and doffing the suit. Traditional dry suits have the zipper located along the back of the shoulder, which requires a buddy to help you put the suit on and take it off. Some suits have front-mounted zippers that allow you to don and doff the suit by yourself and allow for greater torso flexibility.

Most dry suits have a low-pressure inflator and manual and/or automatic exhaust valve. Since the correct operation of the inflator/deflator is critical, you should get professional instruction prior to using the suit in open water. When the suit is not in use, cap the valve of the inflator with a protective nipple to avoid puncturing the suit. All dry suits should have an overexpansion relief valve. On some models, this valve can be adjusted to complement your buoyancy control system.

In addition to a decision regarding the dry suit, you will also need to make a decision regarding the type of underwear to wear under the dry suit. Polypropylene, synthetic pile, radiant insulating garments, and open cell foam are among the more popular materials to be worn under the dry suit. The variety of undergarments along with the variety of dry suits makes it even more important that you purchase your dry suit and accessories only from a professional dive store with a well-established track record in selling dry suits. Because of the rather substantial price involved in the purchase of a dry suit, it is not unreasonable for you to request of the dealer that you be given an opportunity to try out the suit they recommend so that you can get a feel for functioning in the suit before you commit to it.

A period of training is usually required and recommended to gain familiarity with the operation of the valves, additional weighting, and buoyancy control while using the dry suit. In addition, you will wear a buoyancy compensator (BC) with the dry suit because the suit is not suitable as a complete buoyancy control system.

Communication

Since normal talking is usually unintelligible when done underwater, communications consist of hand signals, signs used by the hearing impaired, buddy-line pull signals, light signals, writing messages on a slate, and making noise. There are also some mechanical and electronic devices available that help make normal talking more understandable.

HAND SIGNALS

Divers use three kinds of hand signals: the basic signals, which are generally known throughout the diving community, special signals set by a dive team for use in particular circumstances, and natural signals, which are readily understood anywhere. Figs. 2-7 through 2-30 show samples of various hand signals.

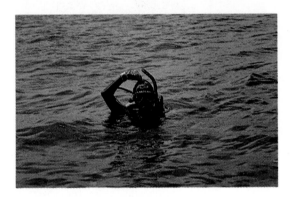

Fig. 2-7 *OK—surface—one arm.*

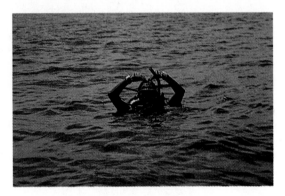

Fig. 2-8 *OK—surface—two arms.*

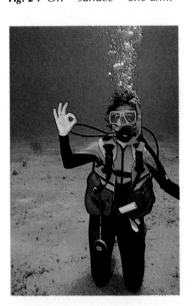

Fig. 2-9 *OK—under—3 sign.*

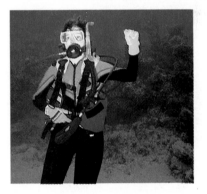

Fig. 2-10 *OK—closed fist.*

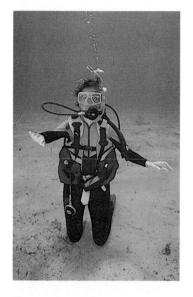

Fig. 2-11 Not OK.

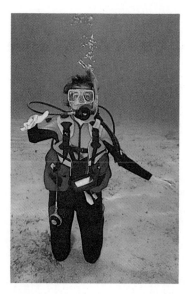

Fig. 2-12 Not OK.

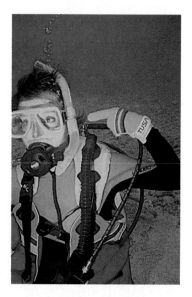

Fig. 2-13 Problem with ears.

Fig. 2-14 Watch.

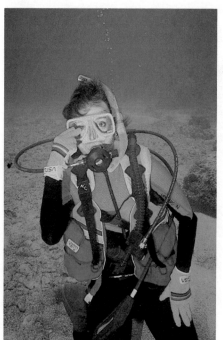

Fig. 2-15 Stop.

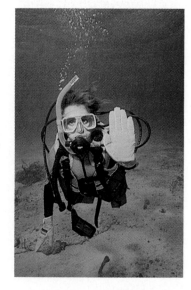

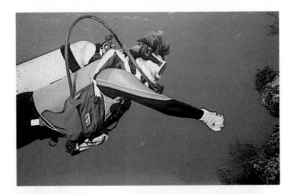

Fig. 2-16 Danger. Closed fist is pointed at object presenting danger.

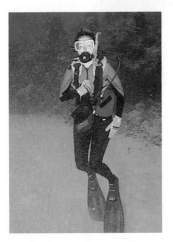

Fig. 2-17 Low on air.

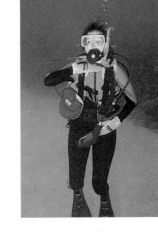

Fig. 2-18 Out of air.

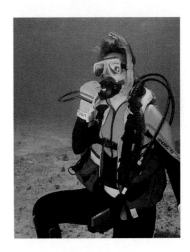

Fig. 2-19 Let's share air.

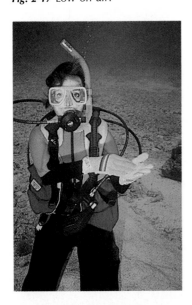

Fig. 2-20 Check air—palm.

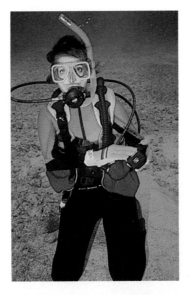

Fig. 2-21 Check air—console.

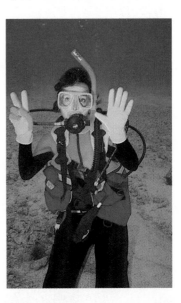

Fig. 2-22 Pounds of air in 100s (700 psi shown).

55

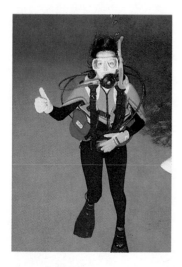

Fig. 2-23 Go up.

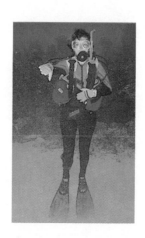

Fig. 2-24 Go down.

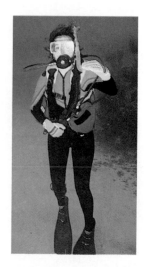

Fig. 2-25 Go over/around/under.

Fig. 2-26 Go this way.

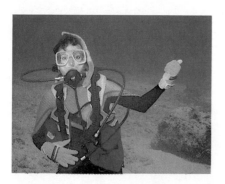

Fig. 2-27 I'm cold.

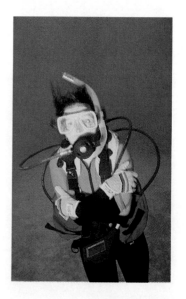

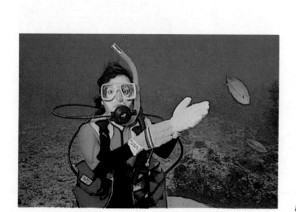

Fig. 2-28 Follow.

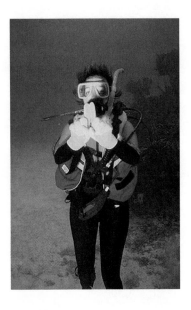

Fig. 2-29 *Get with or closer to buddy.*

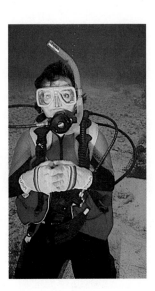

Fig. 2-30 *Boat.*

SIGNS

Use of the Manual Alphabet and manual communication (Figs. 2-31 and 2-32), signs commonly known to hearing-impaired divers, is the closest approximation of talking underwater.

BUDDY-LINE PULL SIGNALS

When a buddy-line is used, pulling it quickly and purposefully about a foot, communicates simple messages as follows:

- Two pulls means "stop," "change direction," or "need more line"
- Three pulls means "come to surface" or "have found object of search"
- Four pulls from diver means "need help"

You may find regional or local variations to pull signals.

LIGHT SIGNALS

Light signals are normally used at night. Flashing the light or shaking its beam in the receiver's field of view means "pay attention to me." Once attention is gained, normal hand signals are used by shining the light on them. Making a big vertical circle slowly indicates "OK."

WRITING MESSAGES ON A SLATE

Writing with a standard wooden pencil on a plastic slate may be tedious, but it can be very precise for detailed messages. In place of a wooden pencil, you might visit an art supply shop and purchase an artist's graphite stick, since the entire object

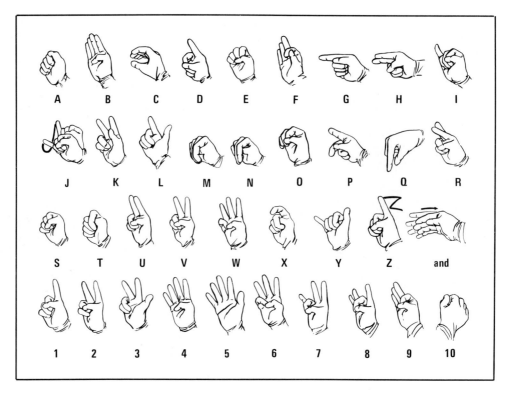

Fig. 2-31 *Manual Alphabet developed as used by the National Association of the Deaf for communication by the hearing impaired.*

can be written with and you will not "break off the point," as sometimes happens with a pencil. The slate is also a good place for recording information regarding the dive profile and observations. A slate can be erased with a standard eraser when the slate is dry, a kitchen abrasive cleanser, or sand. Slates can also have prewritten messages on them to which you simply point.

MAKING NOISE

Making noise by banging a knife on the tank, hooting, shouting, singing, or screaming through the regulator is good only for telling a diver that the signaller wants attention. Since the speed of sound in water is faster than in air it is practically impossible to determine the direction of noise. The receiver will therefore have to search for its source.

ELECTRONIC COMMUNICATORS

Used largely in commercial diving, electronic communicators are available but not widely used in recreational diving.

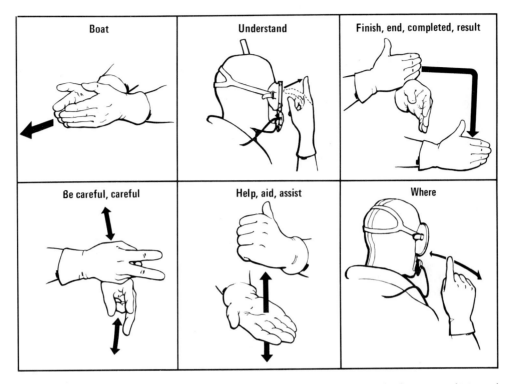

Fig. 2-32 Examples of Manual Communication. A complete book on the language of Manual Communication (the National Association of the Deaf) can be secured by contacting your local center for the hearing impaired.

Some communicators utilize either a throat microphone or a microphone placed inside the mouth. These have two major disadvantages. The throat microphone relies strictly on vibration from the throat into the microphone, which does not permit the necessary quality for real clarity. Placing a microphone inside your mouth and trying to speak around it, particularly while you have a regulator in your mouth as well, can create some rather severe but not insurmountable disadvantages with clarity.

Another electronic communicator, one that requires a special mask with your second-stage regulator installed, permits the microphone to be placed close to the mouth and allows the lips to move freely. You are able to form the words more carefully, and the quality of transmission is significantly improved.

A diving helmet, a device widely used in commercial diving operations, creates an air atmosphere around the head that improves underwater communications in two ways. First, the type of microphone used is superior, and, since you speak into an air atmosphere, the resonance and word formations are vastly improved. The ability to hear is also improved because the sound is transmitted into the air instead of water. The primary problems with this system are its expense, the need for a wire connected to the surface, and the requirement for more sophisticated training.

The basic problem of underwater communication has plagued divers and manufacturers for many years. They are constantly working to improve the quality of mechanical components as well as the standard techniques of underwater communication. There are many possibilities for the future that look promising.

Extended Dives

One continuing desire of divers is to stay down longer. There has been a constant search since the original development of scuba to give the diver longer bottom times, but there still are few options.

One approach to this problem is larger tanks that provide more capacity. These are generally impractical because larger tanks mean increased weight and reduced mobility. A second solution is multiple tanks. If you plan to dive with multiple tanks, you should undergo a period of additional training to become familiar with their assembly and operation. The third option, which is most practical to the sport diver, is higher pressure. The standard 71.2-cubic foot steel tank normally is full at 2475 (its psig plus the 10% overfill) rated 2250 psig and provides about 30 minutes of bottom time for the average diver in less than 33 feet of water. Bottom time, of course, varies with individual breathing rate, activity level, water conditions, depth, physical size, and stress. Also, experienced divers tend to use less air than novice divers. Other normally used cylinders are the 3000 psig models available in the 70, 80, 90, and 100 cubic foot sizes. Also, more recently, steel tanks that handle 3500 psig have become readily available. Although they require a special DIN connector for the first stage regulator because of the high pressures involved, they are available in 65, 80, and 100 cubic foot capacities. From the standpoint of convenience, the 3500-psig 80 is approximately the same size as the steel 55, and the 3500-psig 100 is approximately the same size as the aluminum 80. The diver gains a significant increase in available air without increase in bulk or weight.

There are some small cylinders made in Europe that can hold up to 5000 psig. Cylinders with pressures approaching 5000 psig may be impractical because most air refill stations cannot fill tanks to that high a pressure level. Also, in the United States most regulators are not designed to work with such pressures.

The most common sport diving tanks used today are made of either chrome molybdenum steel or an aluminum alloy. Other alloys, such as the one developed for the 3500-psig tanks, are being introduced into cylinder manufacturing and may ultimately provide even greater options. The newer alloys will continue to allow even more desirable compromises between weight, capacity, length, and diameter, making it easier and easier for the diver to carry cylinders with increased volumes.

Prior to increases in tank capacity, recreational divers were more likely to run out of air than to exceed the no-decompression time limits during nonrepetitive dives of 60 feet or less. However, with current technology, it is possible to extend your dive time to well over an hour. Although this may seem to be a bonus for most divers, it has some drawbacks. When you extend your dive time, you place yourself in a situation where no-decompression diving may be jeopardized. You should always monitor your gauges and accurately calculate your no-decompression time limits during any dive. This essential step becomes increasingly important when you dive with higher capacity tanks.

Surface-Supplied Air

By definition, the scuba diver's air supply is self-contained or limited. For extended bottom times, the scuba diver must carry huge quantities of air in the form of double or even triple tanks. The limiting factor is the physical prowess of the individual diver. Surface-supplied divers, on the other hand, have a virtually unlimited amount of air without the back-breaking weight of multiple tanks (Fig. 2-33). Some surface supply systems available to the recreational diving community can supply more than one diver at a time in shallow water. The limiting factor for the surface-supplied diver is fuel to run the compressor or the amount of air in surface storage cylinders. The best application of this type of technology is to the fields of underwater science and light commercial work. Surface-supplied air is ideal for working divers needing extended bottom times while working in confined areas.

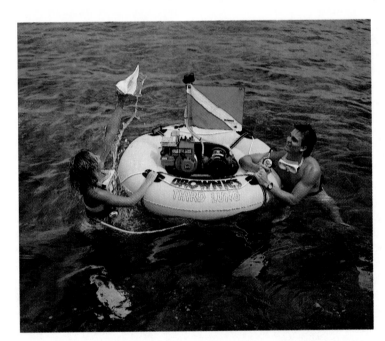

Fig. 2-33 *Surface-supplied air system in use. (Courtesy of Steve Lucas and Brownie's Third Lung.)*

Safety is of significant importance to the tethered, surface-supplied diver. A topside compressor feeding a surface-supply system must have an air reservoir from which the air is drawn for the diver. Without the reservoir, stopping the compressor would result in rapid termination of air flow to the diver below. If the air is supplied to the diver via a full face mask or helmet, the system must have a non-return valve. Failure of the umbilical could result in explosive air loss from the system, causing severe physical injury to the diver's head and face if not protected by a non-return valve. The vast majority of surface-supplied configurations provide the diver with emergency or auxilliary air supplies. The surface-supplied diver can bail

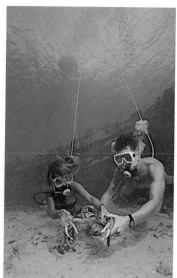

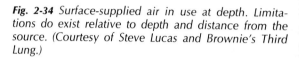

Fig. 2-34 *Surface-supplied air in use at depth. Limitations do exist relative to depth and distance from the source. (Courtesy of Steve Lucas and Brownie's Third Lung.)*

out to a small emergency scuba system that may be integrated into the helmet/mask or regulator system.

There are surface-supplied air systems that actually use a combination of equipment types. Hookah, for example, uses a supply of surface air attached via an umbilical to a scuba regulator on a diver-worn backplate. This technology allows for easy transition for scuba divers to a surface-supplied mode. A hookah-equipped diver needs only a standard scuba mask rather than a full-face mask or helmet (Fig. 2-34).

The major disadvantage of surface-supplied air diving is the loss of true mobility. The umbilical or tether restricts the diver's movement and may make it absolutely necessary to precisely retrace the path to prevent fouling. Fouling of the diver's umbilical may compromise the diver's safety by interfering with the ability to surface in an emergency. Strong currents may create significant resistance to the tethered diver's movement, adding extra work to the dive. There are depth limitations based on the supply abilities available with different types of systems, and extensive surface support may be needed to monitor the surface-supplied diver and air equipment.

Additional Equipment

In addition to items needed for safer, more comfortable, and longer diving, there is equipment that permits you to advance to other areas of interest beyond simply using scuba gear. Propulsion units, underwater metal detectors, and hand-held sonar increase mobility, add significantly to hobbies, or, in some cases, permit safe return to the entry/exit point. Additionally, a relatively new innovation is the alternate second stage that is built into the low-pressure inflator hose on the BC. While there are other items available, these pieces of equipment draw the most practical interest.

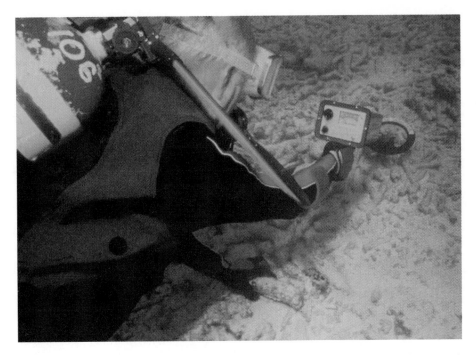

Fig. 2-35 *One of several metal detectors available to scuba divers in use. (Courtesy of JW Fishers.)*

PROPULSION UNITS

Diver propulsion vehicles (DPVs) increase your mobility underwater and can add to the enjoyment of a dive. They have been used in advanced applications to penetrate caves further, increase the range of search and recovery operations, and increase the duration of dives by minimizing the diver's efforts while in the water. They have also been utilized by handicapped divers, allowing them greater mobility and freedom while diving. The vehicles are motor driven and use battery power to move at speeds of from 1 to 3 knots, which is about as fast as you can move comfortably without too much drag on the body. If you turn your head while moving at this speed, the resistance of the water can remove your mask.

Units have variable range and power capabilities. Some larger units and some vehicles with two motors have the capabilities of pulling more than one diver at sustained speeds of 1 to 3 knots. Depending on the battery's size and durability and whether the unit is used continuously or intermittently, propulsion units can run from 1 to 4 hours. Some vehicles with lights integrated into them allow for their use at night. Regardless of the type of vehicle used, all members of the dive team should be equally mobile. It is not a wise practice for one member of a buddy team to use a propulsion vehicle while the other swims. Additional training may be required to use diver propulsion vehicles to learn safety practices particular to those units.

METAL DETECTORS

Several metal detectors are available and, depending on their design, they may detect anything from steel to gold (Fig. 2-35). They can pick up signals from 6 to 12 inches beneath the bottom. Metal detectors work very much like sonar—they send out a pulse that reflects off metal objects. The returning pulse triggers an audible impulse in the metal detector, so you can tell when you have "hit" metal. An increased impulse activity indicates the location and magnitude of the object. Metal detectors can add significantly to the interest of diving and help you locate lost objects and such things as underwater cables or pipelines. These units are relatively inexpensive and can add significantly to the potential joy of diving.

ALTERNATE INFLATION REGULATOR

Alternate inflation regulators, a number of which are now in the marketplace, combine the functions of the inflation/deflation device on the buoyancy control device and the octopus regulator. The alternate inflation regulator is installed on the low pressure inflator/deflator hose of the BC.

The demand regulator is designed for emergency breathing; it is not normally used in place of the primary breathing regulator. It can supplement or replace the octopus regulator, and it can be connected to the main tank or to a separate "pony bottle." To use this regulator in a shared air situation, you give your primary to your buddy and you use the alternate inflation regulator yourself. This device can

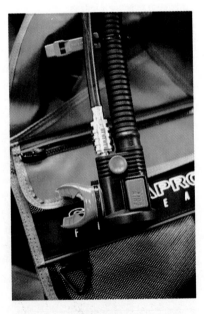

Fig. 2-36 *The alternate inflation regulator can either replace the octopus or serve as a back-up to the octopus.*

be used with a reserve air supply. In both situations, you must have sufficient air capacity, especially at depth (Fig. 2-36).

As recreational diving grows, many such specialty items will be developed to enhance the diver's enjoyment and to provide additional safety. At present, it is enough to have a good understanding of why protection from the cold is so important to your personal comfort, how to add to your safety and enjoyment by monitoring vital information, and how to communicate with your buddy so you are safer and able to share your experience on a moment-to-moment basis. Hopefully, at some point in the future, you may be able to stay down longer to study further or simply enjoy the beauty of the underwater environment. Understanding these things adds to the overall enjoyment and safety of recreational diving.

3 Underwater Photography

At the conclusion of this chapter you should be able to:

1. Describe the simplest form of camera for the beginner that is available at most dive shops and diving resorts.

2. Tell two significant features of a single lens reflex camera that may make it desirable.

3. Name the feature of the single lens reflex camera that is missing in the self-contained underwater camera.

4. Describe the piece of equipment that might be used to accurately assess the amount of light available for underwater photographs.

5. State the approximate depth limitations of disposable or cartridge type underwater cameras.

6. State the depth limitation for less expensive cameras to produce good quality photographs.

7. Name the equipment that is needed to offset the loss of colors at depth.

8. Explain the problems that may lead to "fuzzy" underwater photographs.

9. State which lenses are usually considered wide-angle for underwater photography.

10. State which lenses are usually considered standard lenses for underwater photography.

KEY TERMS

SLR	Refraction	Wide-angle
Standard	Telephoto	Zoom lens
Autofocus lenses	Macro	Video

As your skin diving and scuba experiences broaden, you will probably decide that you would like to find a way to preserve some of the marvelous experiences you have had on your diving adventures. Land photographers who have tried the underwater realm realize that they see substantially more examples of wildlife in one brief dive than they may see in days above the water. Whether you dive in fresh or

67

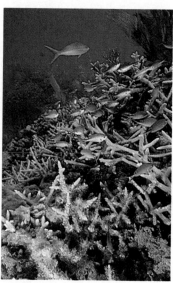

Fig. 3-1 *Divers have found that taking photos while diving is a way to preserve the exciting scenes and events of memorable dives.*

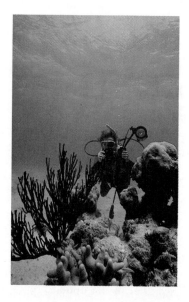

Fig. 3-2 *The basics of underwater photography are not too difficult to master.*

salt water, there is an endless array of photographic subjects that will pass before you (Fig. 3-1).

Most divers who are sensitive to the ecology of fresh waters and the oceans have given up spear fishing. However, the thrill of the stalk and the hunt can be found in the water using the camera. Tremendous skill, talent, and patience are required to "capture" your prey on film (Fig. 3-2).

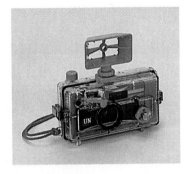

Fig. 3-3 *An inexpensive, entry-level introduction to underwater photography.*

Land Cameras in Housings
DISPOSABLE CAMERAS

At most dive stores, diving resorts, and on liveaboard dive boats you are likely to find disposable cameras available in waterproof housings. These inexpensive cameras enable the diver to try out underwater photography without any investment. Typically, the dive operator sells you the disposable camera and builds into the price the rental of the housing. The entire unit is returned at the end of the dive and your photos are processed. It is doubtful that with such equipment you will produce photos that will appear on the cover of the next issue of your favorite diving magazine, but you will have preserved some memories of your diving experience (Fig. 3-3).

CARTRIDGE AND AUTO 35s WITH HOUSINGS

The next step up in underwater photography is the small 110 or inexpensive 35 mm camera with waterproof housing. Many divers already own such cameras, and if not, these cameras are either available for rent or may be purchased at a price most divers will not find prohibitive. Advantages are that lens selections offer a little better quality than with the disposables, and the diver is buying only film and processing each time diving adventures are recorded. These relatively simple cameras require the same care and handling as more sophisticated cameras. After each dive, the camera housing should be thoroughly washed off in fresh water and allowed to dry before it is opened. Seals and "O" rings require inspection prior to each dive, and appropriate silicone lubricant should be applied as required and consistent with the manufacturer's instructions.

For the diver who is uncertain whether or not underwater photography will be a major activity while diving, the small camera with housing is probably the appropriate "entry level" piece of equipment.

SINGLE LENS REFLEX CAMERAS

The single lens reflex (SLR) camera is probably the most versatile of all cameras available. These cameras feature interchangeable lenses and through-the-lens viewing, allowing you to see the exact image that will appear on the film and to adjust

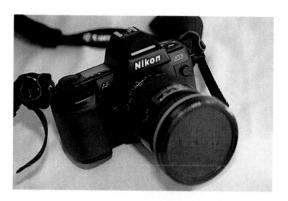

Fig. 3-4 *The SLR has the advantages of flexibility, availability of zoom lenses, and ease of use above or beneath the water.*

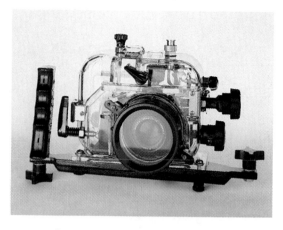

Fig. 3-5 *The SLR in a housing is a very versatile and popular camera arrangement for many underwater photographers. (Courtesy of J. Gale Livers, Ikelite Underwater Systems.)*

the focus accordingly. Supplemented by bulk film magazines, motor drives, and sophisticated data banks that do some of the thinking for the photographer, the SLR is the camera of choice for professionals and talented amateurs (Fig. 3-4).

On the market are a variety of housings that vary from simple sealing "pouches" to the more sophisticated plastic, lexan, and metal housings. Many professional underwater photographers prefer to use housings because they eliminate the need for the purchase of a separate array of underwater cameras and lenses in addition to the land photographic equipment they already utilize. See Fig. 3-5 for an example of the housed SLR camera.

Self-Contained Underwater Cameras

For photographers who do not wish to expose their expensive cameras to the underwater elements (it is a rare, experienced underwater photographer who has not flooded a camera or housing at least once), the self-contained underwater camera is the choice. These cameras are quite expensive, but several companies have introduced more reasonably priced units to the market in recent years.

Although lacking the through-the-lens viewing of the SLR, the self-contained unit offers significant advantages to the underwater photographer. These cameras are ruggedly constructed and able to withstand the rigors of diving. They offer a relatively wide variety of lenses, automatic features to adjust shutter speed, close-up attachments and extension tubes for macrophotography, and flash units that are not only synchronized but adjust flash intensity based on the amount of light entering the lens. Producing extremely high quality photographs, these are the cameras used by many professionals. The only significant disadvantage of self-contained units is the need to estimate distance and the inability to see through the viewfinder to check if your subject is in focus (Fig. 3-6).

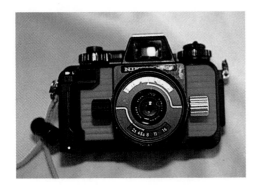

Fig. 3-6 *A popular self-contained underwater camera.*

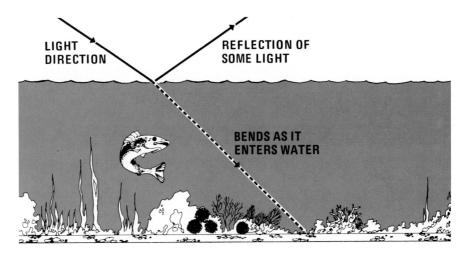

Fig. 3-7 *Water reflects, absorbs, and bends natural light.*

Natural Light Photography Underwater
PROBLEMS FOR BEGINNERS

Light

Photography underwater is much more difficult than on land. Water bends and absorbs light rays, as you can see in Fig. 3-7. Wave action reflects a significant amount of available light and reduces the amount available to illuminate your subject. Since your brain has the remarkable ability to adjust for changes in light intensity, it is less noticeable to the diver that there is substantially less light in the water than on the surface.

The bending of light in water, refraction, is a problem that is partially offset by the fields-of-view of the "standard" underwater lens. For land photography, the 50 mm lens is considered a "standard," but in the water 35 mm or 28 mm is a "standard." The wider angle of view provided by these lenses with shorter focal lengths (the distance indicated by the millimeter identification) in part corrects for the water's refraction. However, most beginners are disappointed by their first underwater photographic efforts. First, objects they thought would fill the photograph appear quite small—this is one effect of refraction. Second, it is not unusual to see pictures underexposed or overexposed as the beginner estimates available light or as light intensities change. Rather than guessing, many experienced underwater photographers invest in underwater light meters to confirm their "guesstimates." This might be a useful purchase if you wish to seriously pursue underwater photography.

As a simple rule of thumb, disposable or cartridge type cameras are probably only effective in clear water to a depth of not much beyond 15 feet. Less expensive alternative cameras may perform satisfactorily to depths of around 30 feet in good conditions. Beyond those limitations, it takes relatively expensive equipment to achieve good results.

Color

Many beginners find that there is little color in their photographs and wonder why their pictures of a given fish or sponge did not possess the same vivid colors as seen in the photos taken by the "pros." The answer quite simply is the absorption of color at depth and the need for artificial illumination to offset the color loss (Fig. 3-8). Reds begin to disappear almost immediately and are gone at around 16 feet; by 33 feet oranges are gone, followed by yellows and greens. In spite of the fact that some yellows remain, below 33 feet everything takes on a blue-green cast. By the time one reaches a depth of 60 feet, the only colors usually captured on film in natural light will be blue to violet hues and grays, but this is affected by light intensity and water clarity to some extent.

Another factor that will affect color as well as clarity of the photograph is particulate matter in the water. Sediment or organic matter will tend to diminish the clarity and "smudge" the colors in your photos.

For natural light photography in the water to show colors, it is necessary to stay at relatively shallow depths and get as close to your subject as possible.

Artificial Light Photography

The need for an artificial light source becomes obvious as you read the previous paragraphs. At increasing depth, both light and colors are lost. By using an artificial light source that comes close in intensity and quality to that produced by natural light, it is possible to produce photographs of startling quality.

Many of the inexpensive cameras discussed in this section come with built-in flash units that will adequately illuminate subjects at shallower depths and relatively close to the photographer. At greater depths and for artificially lighting subjects at greater distances, it becomes necessary to use far more powerful flash units, the cost of which become relatively prohibitive to the photographer not wishing to become deeply involved in underwater photographic pursuits. Examples of these underwater flash (strobe) units are illustrated in Fig. 3-9.

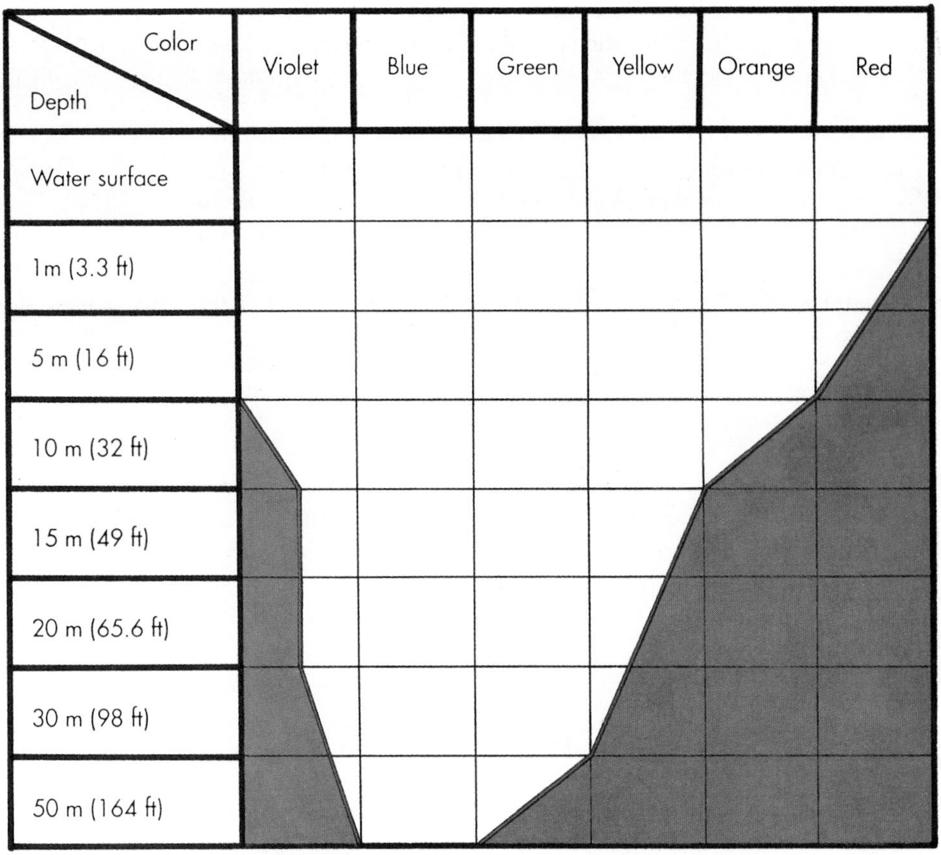

Color \ Depth	Violet	Blue	Green	Yellow	Orange	Red
Water surface						
1m (3.3 ft)						
5 m (16 ft)						
10 m (32 ft)						
15 m (49 ft)						
20 m (65.6 ft)						
30 m (98 ft)						
50 m (164 ft)						

Fig. 3-8 *This is the way that various colors progressively disappear at depth in water.*

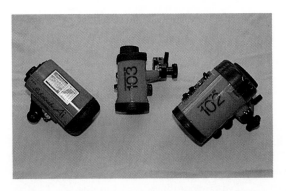

Fig. 3-9 *Representative artificial light sources most popular in underwater photography.*

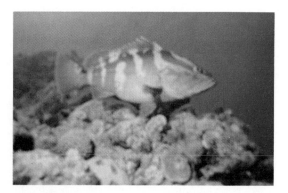

Fig. 3-10 *This is how your pictures may appear secondary to the camera movement. Notice that everything in the photograph appears to be "fuzzy."*

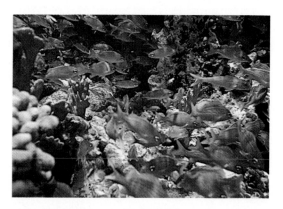

Fig. 3-11 *If the subject or portion of your subject appears "fuzzy," this is usually the result of subject movement. To avoid this problem, use the fastest possible lens speed appropriate for the flash or amount of available light.*

MOVEMENT

Probably the most common problem encountered by beginning underwater photographers is movement. "Fuzzy" photographs are usually the result of movement . . . either of the camera or the subject.

Elimination of camera movement can be somewhat resolved by assuring that your camera is neutrally buoyant. Otherwise, the only solution is to practice or, as it is described in the photography business, "burn" a lot of film. With time the photographer develops techniques to keep as still as possible. Historically, many photographers used excessive weight to maintain their stability. We now know that many diving deaths are attributable to the use of excessive weight and the inability of the diver to ditch the weight belt in the event of emergency; *photographers should not excessively over-weight for the sake of steadiness!*

Another practice of some photographers in the past has been to hold their breath to steady themselves. If you find it necessary to pause in your breathing cycle when taking a photo, be sure to relax and not ascend. Photographers sometimes find that getting their elbows on the sandy bottom or kneeling on the sandy bottom may assist in stabilizing themselves.

To identify whether it was you or your subject that caused the blurriness that appears in your pictures, check to see if the entire picture is blurred. If it is all blurred then the movement was on the part of the photographer (Fig. 3-10). If, however, the subject is the only thing in the picture that is blurred then the blurriness is the result of subject movement (Fig. 3-11). Eliminating your own movement when photographing is a matter of a firm grip on the camera, having yourself neutrally buoyant, and doing your photography in relatively calm diving conditions. Eliminating blurring due to subject movement is a matter of shutter speed and your position relative to the object. If you pursue underwater photography further,

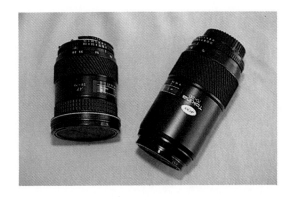

Fig. 3-12 *The zoom lens of the SLR can offer the photographer a great deal of flexibility from wide-angle to close-up capability.*

you will learn about shutter speed, depth of field, and aperture. The key to crisply freezing your subject's movement is to utilize the fastest shutter speed possible compatible with a lens opening that will provide you with adequate light and sufficient depth of field.

Because of the speed with which underwater strobe units fire, many times your subject will be "frozen" in the light of the underwater strobe, and this too is a way that underwater movement can be eliminated as a problem in your photography.

INTERCHANGEABLE LENSES

Whether talking about underwater or terrestrial photography, the general terms relative to lenses are the same: wide-angle, standard, and telephoto.

When using housed SLR cameras, the photographer has the option of using a zoom lens. The zoom lens, shown in Fig. 3-12, varies in focal length and can give the diver a wide variety of lens lengths and thus tremendous versatility with a single lens. However, because of the way that zoom and autofocus lenses work in concert with their cameras, it may be necessary to add a screw-on close-up lens to the zoom lens before installing the camera in its housing. Some of the modern zoom lenses even offer the possibility of doing close-up or macrophotography without changing lenses.

Wide-angle lenses for self-contained underwater cameras are either single lenses or adapters that can be added to standard underwater lenses. Wide-angle lenses are utilized in taking shots of groups of divers, large schools of fish, or underwater scenic shots. Typically the 15 mm or 20 mm lenses are viewed as wide-angle lenses underwater. Additionally, slip-on lens adapters are available that can make a standard lens function in the same manner as a 15 mm lens as far as angle of view is concerned. One of the remarkable attributes of the wide-angle lens is its tremendous depth of field. Using the 15 mm lens, for example, with the appropriate lens opening, everything between a distance of just under 2 feet to infinity is in focus. Though not absolutely necessary, with wide-angle lenses it is best to use a viewfinder that is optically corrected so you can see approximately the same thing that will be captured through the lens. The 15 mm lens with accompanying finder is a

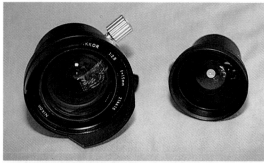

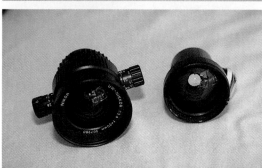

Fig. 3-13 *The wide-angle lenses offer the ability to take beautiful scenic type shots and give the photographer a tremendous depth of field.*

major investment, often two or three times the price of the camera! The 20 mm lens is significantly less expensive and is probably sufficient as a wide-angle lens for most underwater photographers except for professionals and the most serious of amateurs (Fig. 3-13).

The standard lenses are generally viewed as the 28 mm and 35 mm lenses. Because of the impact of refraction, focal lengths are somewhat shorter than the typical 50 mm or 60 mm "standard" lens for land photography. These lenses also use finders, as do their wide-angle cousins, but this may simply be the camera viewfinder, a sight-through framer, or an adaptation of the optical finder for a wide-angle lens. These lenses offer tremendous versatility by making available to the underwater photographer the ability to take slightly narrower field-of-view wide-angle shots as well as relatively close-up fish, animal, and reef shots (Fig. 3-14).

The telephoto lens for the self-contained underwater camera is the 80 mm lens. Using this lens, the photographer can capture from quite a distance shots that might be impossible were the photographer closer to and frightening the subject. This lens has the flexibility to be used above the water as well as underwater (Fig. 3-15).

Close-up and macrophotographs are made with self-contained cameras using either a close-up attachment or extension tubes. Combining various lenses with the close-up lens attachment or a variety of extension tubes enables the photographer to capture some of the beauty found in the smaller aspects of underwater life. Due

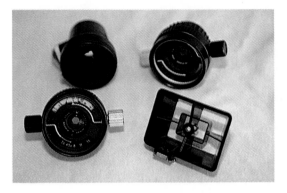

Fig. 3-14 *Examples of two standard lenses and finders.*

Fig. 3-15 *The 80 mm lens is the telephoto lens for underwater use.*

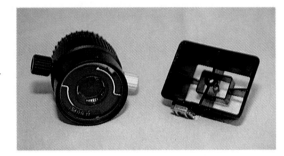

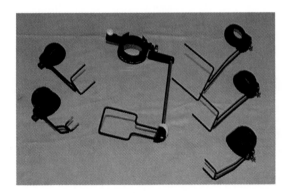

Fig. 3-16 *The extension tubes and close-up attachments enable the photographer to put onto film the beauty and detail of many underwater creatures.*

to an extremely limited depth of field with these devices, the framers enable the photographer to place the subject precisely within the depth of field and thereby capture very sharp close-up photos. Quite often, the beauty and detail present in underwater life is not noticeable until one views the photograph of some underwater life-form whose details were not noticeable when first viewed with the naked eye (Fig. 3-16).

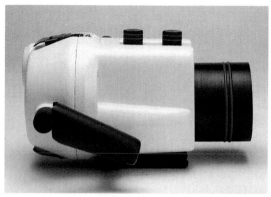

Fig. 3-17 *Modern video housings combined with evolving video technology enable the diver to videotape many underwater adventures without the need for taking bulky equipment in the water. (Courtesy of J. Gale Livers, Ikelite Underwater Systems.)*

Underwater Video

Early efforts at recording diving activities in motion were limited to motion picture film and relatively sophisticated equipment. Early video equipment was extremely heavy and cumbersome; the earliest underwater video systems weighed in at around 100 pounds! With the evolution of videotaping equipment in the 1980s, this medium became more and more available to the diver willing to make the rather significant expenditure involved. However, the technology was still rather limited, and rather bulky equipment was required with substantial accessory lighting needed. Today, as the equipment has evolved further, high-intensity lighting is more compact, and video cameras and their accompanying housings are easier to handle (Fig. 3-17).

The evolutionary process of video has progressed to where the diver has a choice of VHS or Beta formats or the newer, even more compact, 8 mm video format. Fig. 3-18 illustrates a popular video housing using either VHS or Beta format units. To make specific video recommendations in a book such as this would be inappropriate because of the speed with which the video industry develops better and better products. Before getting involved in underwater video, consult with a dive store professional knowledgeable in the video field.

With the quality of video equipment now available, the diver can produce on videotape products that challenge in quality the finest 35 mm still photographs. Video can be used to tape general diving activities that you wish to recall in the future, shoot striking macros, or, with appropriate planning and preparation, tell a story or provide a useful supplement for education or training.

Even if you do not wish to get into videotaping dives on your own, you should consider having a memorable dive videotaped by a professional on a dive trip since it will be a record of that special dive that you will be able to view time and time again. If videotaping dive activities is something that interests you, more dive professionals are now offering training and equipment for you to engage in this activity.

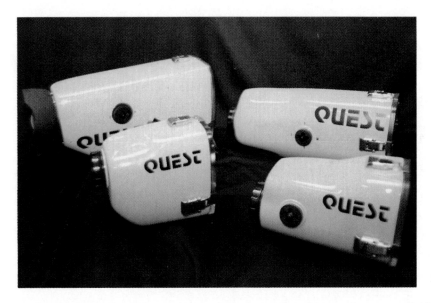

Fig. 3-18 *Another example of the modern variety of compact video equipment available to today's scuba diver. Equipment of this sort both simplifies the video process and makes video as accessible to the diver as is still underwater photography. (Courtesy of Quest Marine Video.)*

Learning Underwater Photography and Video

Nearly all the major diving agencies have specialty courses in underwater photography or video where you will be able to learn this craft from very experienced instructors. In these courses you will be able to use a variety of underwater photographic or video equipment and have an opportunity to "try before you buy." On staff at many dive resorts throughout the world are talented professional underwater photographers and videographers who will share with you their secrets of capturing the underwater world on film or tape. Though the additional expense may at first seem prohibitive, the money you save on wasted film, the rapidity with which you will begin producing "pro-quality" results, and the elimination of the frustration of learning the skill "the hard way" will make the expense seem relatively insignificant.

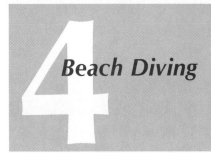

Beach Diving

OBJECTIVES

At the conclusion of this chapter you should be able to:

1. Explain the necessary precautions for beach diving.

2. Describe the use of a diving float when beach diving and why it is necessary.

3. Explain the components of a good emergency plan relative to beach diving activities.

4. Tell what should be consulted before beach diving in areas where tides may have a significant impact on diving safety.

5. Tell how rip currents can be identified.

6. Describe what is meant by wave "sets."

7. Explain two entry methods that may be used in beach diving.

8. State the safety measures to utilize when exiting in rough surf conditions.

9. Describe the fin removal technique that may be utilized when using a crawling exit through heavy surf.

10. Tell how and when you should attempt to stand with your buddy when exiting through rough surf.

KEY TERMS

Tarp	Tide tables	Low impact beach
High impact beach	Rip currents	Long-shore currents
Surf zone		

More and more people each year are finding that diving from the beach is both fun and economical. Divers and their nondiving friends can enjoy a camping trip together to the coast, since the beach can be enjoyed even if you do not dive. Your diving experience can be shared with friends. They can snorkel or explore tidal pools or flats while you dive. Remember that the beaches are for everyone. Try to minimize your impact by leaving the beach cleaner than you found it.

Beach diving is the least expensive, because divers can generally drive to the site in their own vehicles and have only the expenses of gas, parking, gear rental,

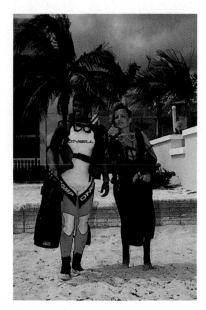

Fig. 4-1 *Two divers set out for a beach dive, probably the most common form of ocean diving in the United States.*

and air. Planning a beach dive can be as simple as agreeing on a location and picking up your buddy or meeting your buddy at the site. With a little forethought, beach diving can be safe and fun. Divers on the west coast of the United States tend to be more comfortable with beach diving and rough surf conditions than those on the east coast. First, west coast divers do much more beach diving than eastern divers, who favor boat-diving. Second, the surf conditions on the west coast tend to be rougher, and year-round water temperatures require diving in more cumbersome equipment than divers from the east who have limited beach diving and tend to be warm-weather beach divers (Fig. 4-1).

Equipment

In addition to your normal scuba dive gear, you may want to pack a few extra items to make your diving day more enjoyable. A plastic bin or bag for wet dive gear to keep your car clean and dry is ideal. A separate ice chest can be carried for drinks and food, along with a tarp or towels to lay on the beach. The tarp or towels will keep sand out of dive equipment (Fig. 4-2). While approaching and walking along the beach, it is important to prevent your equipment from dragging in the sand. This cannot be overemphasized. Sand packed in the second stage of a regulator may cause it to free flow and may require disassembly and cleaning by a qualified technician (Figs. 4-3 and 4-4).

While heavy surf conditions and areas of boat traffic, especially fishing boats trolling in shallow waters, should be avoided, a dive flag on a float should be taken with you to alert boaters of your presence. The float should be trailed behind you as you move through the surf.

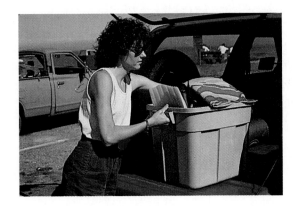

Fig. 4-2 *It is a good idea to take a box in which to store your clothing and gear for the day and a tarp or towel on which to spread out gear. This prevents sand from getting into dive gear. (Courtesy of Matt McDermott.)*

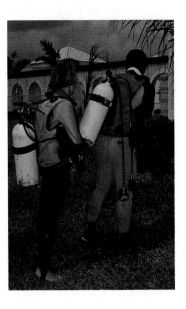

Fig. 4-3 *One approach, where beach access is relatively easy and not too far distant, is to don scuba gear before getting onto the sand. This will prevent sand from getting into your gear.*

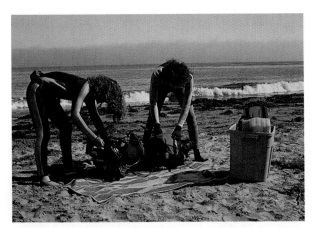

Fig. 4-4 *Where getting to the beach is more difficult, gearing up can take place on the beach, but buddies must be cognizant of gear staying clear of the sand. (Courtesy of Matt McDermott.)*

Dive Planning

If you live some distance from your planned dive site, call ahead to confirm the conditions. Most dive stores and many state parks will be more than happy to give you a weather report at a minimum and some will even provide you with the water conditions.

A good emergency plan is essential. Before leaving for the dive site, let a friend or family member know where you will be diving and your expected time of return. Include in the information communicated where you will park your car and any alternate dive site you may choose if you do not use your first choice. Take along spare change and check the function of any pay phones in the area. (*Note:* In areas served by 911 service, no money is required to place emergency calls, but the phone must be working.) If you will be diving in a remote location, take along essential first aid supplies and oxygen and be sure you can describe your exact location should you require help in the event of an emergency.

In areas where tides can dramatically affect diving conditions, you should check tide tables prior to your dive day to determine the best time to dive. If the area is new to both you and your buddy, consult a local dive store or other source of reliable dive information. They may be able to tell you the most convenient places to park, camp, and dive; what to avoid; where to enter and exit the water and rinse equipment; and where good restaurants are located. This information is free for the asking and can often make the difference between a good and a poor dive trip.

Assessing beach conditions is not difficult. A few minutes of careful observation can help you decide on the best entry and exit points, the mode of entry, and what types of currents you may encounter.

High- and Low-Impact Beaches

Beaches can be broadly divided into two major classes; high and low impact. A low-impact beach usually has little surf action. The sand is generally very fine. In contrast, a high-impact beach has very coarse grained sand or is mostly rocky and uneven. You will often encounter large waves and heavy surf on a high-impact beach, although on calm days or in the morning a normally high-impact beach can offer great diving. Many times, rocky or coral reefs lie a very short distance from both sand and rocky beaches. They can be detected on the west coast by the presence of a kelp bed, or on the east coast by a white water "boil" just off the beach. This white water is caused by a rock or coral reef just below the water's surface. These areas offer outstanding diving opportunities since they shelter myriad forms of marine life.

Currents

Rip currents can be a nuisance if they go undetected. Usually a rip current can be identified by an area of apparently calm water in a region of surf. Actually, water is being channeled out from the beach and under cutting the incoming waves, causing them to lose power and "lay down." While a rip current can move you quickly away from the shore during an entry, this can be deceptive when choosing an exit point, as swimming against a rip can prove tiring and unproductive. If you find yourself in a rip current and making no progress, swim across it, perpendicular to the current, until you are in water that is moving toward the beach.

Long-shore currents should be considered also. These currents, while gentle in some areas, can cause a diver to drift quite a distance from the entry point. If you perceive that you are drifting, you may want to surface to get your bearings before continuing the dive.

Entries

Entries and exits for diving from beaches require careful timing to be most effective. Prior to entering the water you should watch the waves. Generally, there will be a series of smaller waves followed by larger waves in a regularly repeating pattern called *sets*. By watching several of these sets, you can count on the small waves to appear at regular intervals. Begin your entry at the end of the big set to maximize the amount of time available to enter the water.

Depending on the size of the surf and your skill level, you may choose one of two entry methods. For large surf or rocky, uneven beaches, you and your buddy can support one another as you don your fins before entering the water; stand up and use what some divers describe as the "figure-four" technique for fin donning— right hand to don the left fin, and left hand to don the right fin (Fig. 4-5). Once your fins are on and all of your equipment is in place, begin to walk sideways, if surf conditions permit, always keeping an eye on the incoming surf. Walking in

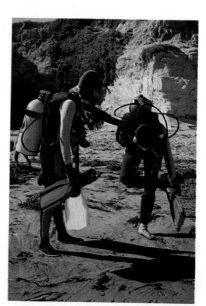

Fig. 4-5 *Where ocean conditions are too rough to permit donning fins in the water, the fins are donned on the beach. (Courtesy of Matt McDermott.)*

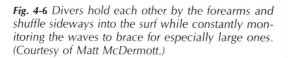

Fig. **4-6** *Divers hold each other by the forearms and shuffle sideways into the surf while constantly monitoring the waves to brace for especially large ones. (Courtesy of Matt McDermott.)*

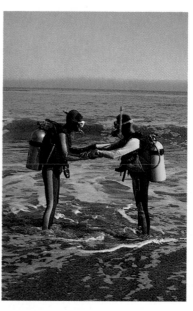

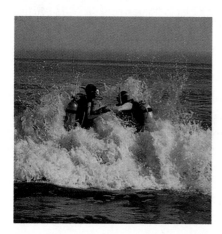

Fig. **4-7** *If divers are hit by a wave, they are bracing each other. This will prevent them from being rolled over by the wave. (Courtesy of Matt McDermott.)*

sideways presents a relatively small surface area to the incoming surf (Fig. 4-6). In particularly heavy surf, a sideways entry may lead to being spun by the surf and backing in may be superior—meeting force with force or diving under the surf. When backing into a heavy surf, keep a constant watch on the waves. Bend your knees so you can remain stable, and stop walking and brace yourself with a wide stance as the waves break around you. If necessary, maintain contact with your buddy by holding hands to help stabilize each other; at the same time, maintain control of your mask (Fig. 4-7).

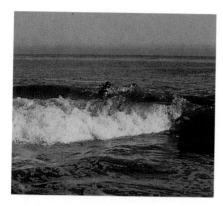

Fig. 4-8 *Once in water that is deep enough, the divers turn into the waves and swim through them until they are clear of the surf zone. (Courtesy of Matt McDermott.)*

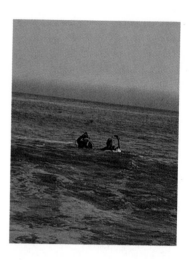

Fig. 4-9 *Once clear of the surf zone, the divers turn and give the "OK" signal back to the beachmaster or divemaster. (Courtesy of Matt McDermott.)*

Once in thigh-deep water or if you should fall, you should turn and swim out under and through the incoming waves (Figs. 4-8 and 4-9). You can control your mask when going under the surf by placing one hand on it. If the worst happens and you get tumbled by the waves, do not panic. With your regulator in your mouth, you have all the air you need. You need to decide whether you will swim out through the waves or crawl back out up the beach. While moving through the surf, remember to keep your gear out of the sand. Also, keep in mind that a regulator in the mouth and big surf hold the same potential for an embolism as being submerged—Boyle's Law still applies once the water gets deeper, so maintain control and do not hold your breath in the surf. Do not attempt to stand up in a rough surf with your fins on. Crawling can be faster, safer, and much more effective.

On low surf beaches, entries are much easier. You may decide to wade in to waist deep water before donning your fins. You can then lean on your buddy or float while putting them on. Then roll and swim out (Figs. 4-10 to 4-12).

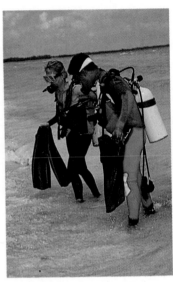

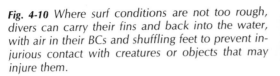

Fig. 4-10 Where surf conditions are not too rough, divers can carry their fins and back into the water, with air in their BCs and shuffling feet to prevent injurious contact with creatures or objects that may injure them.

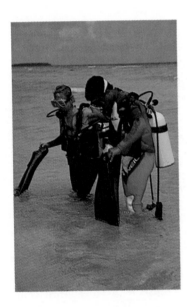

Fig. 4-11 The divers continue to back into the water while watching the wave set for any waves that might knock the divers off their feet. Notice that this buddy pair is steadying each other during the entry.

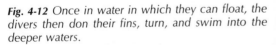

Fig. 4-12 Once in water in which they can float, the divers then don their fins, turn, and swim into the deeper waters.

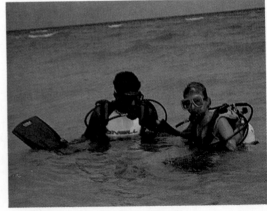

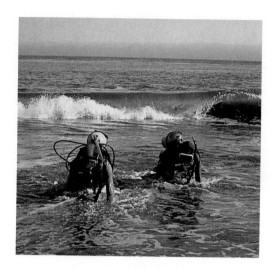

Fig. 4-13 When exiting through a rough surf, divers should keep their regulators in place, fins on, and crawl once they are on beach surface. (Courtesy of Matt McDermott.)

Fig. 4-14 Once in an area where fin removal appears to be safe, the trailing diver kneels on her buddy's fins and removes the fins from behind. The role is then reversed as the trailing diver crawls by the leading diver. (Courtesy of Matt McDermott.)

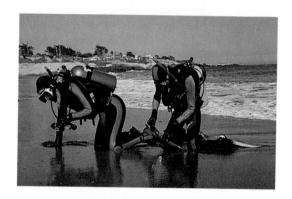

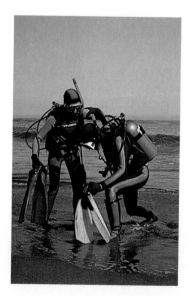

Fig. 4-15 While continuing to watch for big waves, the dive buddies help each other up after fins have been removed and walk from the zone of the beach where waves may present any risk. (Courtesy of Matt McDermott.)

Fig. 4-16 When exiting through a gentle surf, the buddy pair swims until it reaches a place where both buddies can stand and steady one another.

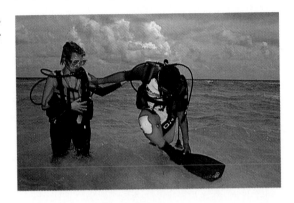

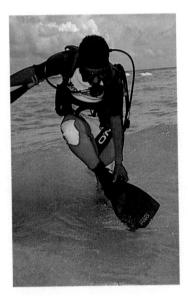

Fig. 4-17 Then, while the support for each other continues, the fins are removed and the divers can walk out of the water.

Exits

Exits are easier than entries. Begin by watching the surf from just beyond the surf zone to determine when it is calm and safe to exit. With your regulator in your mouth and your console and alternate air source tucked safely in your buoyancy compensator (BC), start in to the beach as the last large wave of the set passes and swim until you can begin to crawl. The incoming water will help you up the beach. Then brace yourself or "dig in" to prevent losing ground to the backwash. Continue to crawl as soon as you are able. Get clear of the surf zone as soon as possible because it is here where you can get tumbled by waves (Fig. 4-13). Once you and your buddy have crawled clear of the water, have your buddy crawl in front of you and stop. Kneel on your buddy's fins and remove the straps while having your buddy crawl out of the fins. Put your hands through the straps so as not to lose them in the surf. Next, crawl in front of your buddy and repeat the process (Fig. 4-14). You can now help each other to stand (Fig. 4-15). In calm conditions, you may be able to swim in, remove your fins, and walk out without crawling (Figs. 4-16 and 4-17).

5 Boat Diving

OBJECTIVES

At the conclusion of this chapter you should be able to:

1. Describe how a dive boat can provide you with a base of operations and how it can be utilized in that manner.

2. Describe the general types of dive boat that may be used by scuba divers.

3. Explain the factors that should be considered in choosing a commercial dive boat.

4. Tell the differences between large dive boats and those that carry six or fewer passengers.

5. Name the vital equipment that should be found on all dive boats.

6. Regardless of the size of the dive boat, name the equipment that should be on board for the possible care of injured divers.

7. State several sources you may utilize to get information regarding dive boat operators and dive boat trips.

8. Name the piece of equipment to be utilized on a dive boat to keep your equipment organized and stored compactly.

9. Explain the types of meals that should be consumed before going on a dive boat trip.

10. Describe how best to deal with motion sickness on board a dive boat.

KEY TERMS

Live-aboard	Forward	Aft
Bilge	Bulkheads	Ladders
Overhead	Galley	Head
Fathom	Leeward	Windward
Roll	Pitching	Yaw
PFD	Oxygen equipment	Gear bag
Giant stride entry	Back roll entry	Tag line
U.S.C.G. Auxiliary	U.S. Power Squadron	Mooring

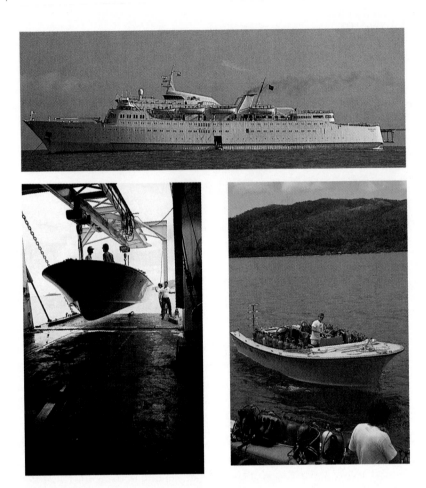

Fig. 5-1 *Boat diving can be as grand as a cruise ship designed exclusively for diving.*

Diving from boats has been part of recreational diving since the beginning. Now, it is one of the fastest-growing activities. Charter or commercial dive boats are used in diving areas where no boats were previously found. More boats operate in established boat diving areas and these are becoming larger and better equipped, with many built strictly for diving. Luxury "live-aboard" dive boats are becoming very-popular. These floating dive hotels can take guests to very remote dive destinations for several days at a time, offering nearly unlimited diving on virgin reefs, and providing open water and advanced certifications while on board (Fig. 5-1). At the same time, more divers are using private boats (Fig. 5-2).

Divers now ask for more and better services, and diving instruction, techniques, and equipment have improved to the point that it is worthwhile to build and operate both large and small dive boats. These improved boats give divers a taste of the ease and fun of boat diving and, in turn, stimulate increased diving in general.

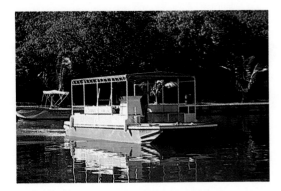

Fig. 5-2 This is a smaller pontoon dive boat operating in the Caribbean.

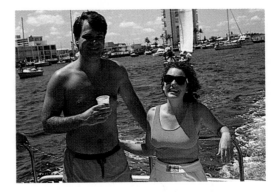

Fig. 5-3 Boat diving can be an extremely pleasant way to dive, and you may strike up new friendships.

The dive boat provides a base of operations where you can rest, change gear, eat, get warm, and talk. This contributes to the safety, security, ease, comfort, and the very joy of diving. Boat diving lets you dive in areas where it would not otherwise be possible, and at the same time, lets you enjoy diving activities not possible from the shore (Fig. 5-3).

In some areas, boats are often the only way to dive in water that is calm, clear, or deep. It is best to do night diving from a boat. Hunting, collecting, wreck diving, underwater photography, search and recovery, light salvage, and drift diving are all best done from a boat. Boats also provide a social aspect to diving—an opportunity to interact with fellow divers who share this common interest.

Yet, with all that boat diving has to offer, there are still possible difficulties. You may have had no preparation for boat diving during your training. You may have been on small, uncomfortable boats in the past. You may not know how to find a dive boat or how to act when on board. You may be concerned about getting seasick. All these are reasonable concerns because they interfere with safe, comfortable, and enjoyable diving.

This chapter provides you with information about the characteristics of dive boats, how to find a dive boat, how to prepare for a boat dive, making your boat dive more enjoyable, specific boat diving techniques, and how to conduct diving activities from your own boat.

Dive Boats
TYPES

Charter or commercial dive boats are businesses that provide diving trips. These boats vary greatly in size, arrangement, and equipment, but are similar to sport fishing boats. The first dive boats were converted from sport fishing or military boats. Now boats are often built specifically for diving, but the hull and superstructure will still resemble fishing boats. In some areas, where less boat diving is done, boats may alternate between carrying divers and fishermen.

Private boats used for diving may be any type or size. Large luxury yachts, cabin cruisers, sailboats, open outboards, and inflatable boats are all used. Small open boats with outboard motors, including both inflatables, and hard materials, such as wood, metal, and fiberglass, have become the most popular private boats for diving. Inflatable boats are easy to transport and can be used almost anywhere. Small boats are less expensive, easier to maneuver and dive from, and most often faster than large boats. Small boats usually need very few modifications for diving. Additionally, kayaks are now being designed with the diver in mind. These "sit on" type ocean kayaks are designed with flotation and storage capacity for a diver and dive gear. Kayaks are light and portable. They are becoming very popular for divers who want to reach offshore diving without having to swim or incur the expense of a larger boat.

Another category of surface support includes surface floats, such as inner tubes, surf mats, paddleboards, surfboards, and other flotation devices built especially for divers. These floats are valuable safety tools for divers. They are not actually boats, but they do provide some of the same advantages, such as a place to rest, store extra gear, adjust gear, discuss the dive, and make rescues. These surface floats are most often used on dives made from shore, but they also may be used from boats. Using floats may help to keep from moving the boat or they may be used to increase your range of activities.

Parts of a Boat

You will naturally be more comfortable on a boat if you know the names and appearance of different parts and equipment. Figs. 5-4 and 5-5 show the general parts of a boat; Fig. 5-6 indicates the general layout for a dive boat.

When you face the bow, you are said to be facing forward. Turning around and facing the stern, you are facing aft. The bilge is the lower inside area of the hull. Bulkheads are the walls, the deck is the floor, ladders are steps, and the overhead is the ceiling. The galley is the kitchen and the head is the bathroom.

An anchor is a specially-shaped metal device designed to dig into the bottom underwater and hold the boat in place. A mooring is a semipermanent anchorage with a heavy anchor, chain, buoy, and line.

A fathom is a measure of length used on boats and in the water. It is equal to 6 feet. The direction away from the wind is called leeward, and windward means facing into the wind. The sideways rotational motion of a boat is called roll, while the vertical rise and fall of the bow is called pitching. Yaw is when the bow falls off course to either side.

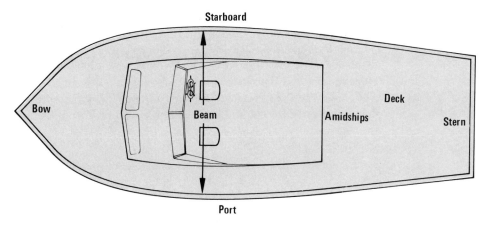

Fig. 5-4 *Top view of boat.*

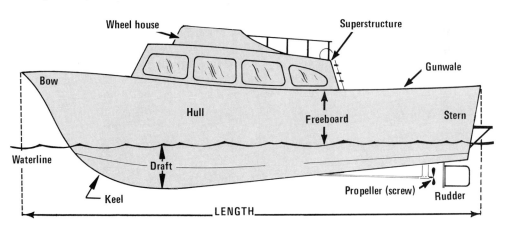

Fig. 5-5 *Side view of boat.*

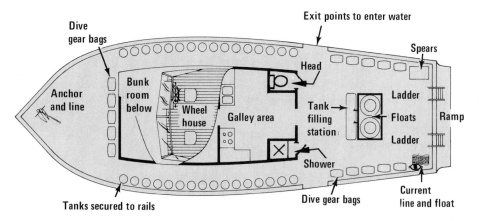

Fig. 5-6 *Top view of one type of commercial dive boat with features that will be found on most dive boats identified.*

COMMERCIAL BOAT DIVING

Most diving is done from commercial dive boats. You may choose to dive from a small or large commercial dive boat. There are several things to consider before selecting the type of boat from which you want to dive. These include licensing of both the boat and the operator, type of equipment available, and activities offered in the area the boat is going. Be sure any boat you choose is properly set up for diving, otherwise, it could turn out to be a difficult day of diving.

COAST GUARD REQUIREMENTS

When diving in or from the United States, you should not go on a boat diving trip unless certain U.S. Coast Guard requirements are met. These requirements are your assurance that the boat is safe and has proper equipment, and that the operator is qualified (Fig. 5-7). Most foreign countries have no requirements, so, when boat diving in foreign waters, you should do your own thorough safety check.

U.S. Coast Guard requirements create two distinct categories of boats. Large boats that carry more than six passengers for hire are required to have both the boat and operator licensed by the Coast Guard. A passenger for hire is any person who has contributed anything directly or indirectly for the passage. This could be money, food, gas, and so forth. Any operator should be knowledgeable about boats

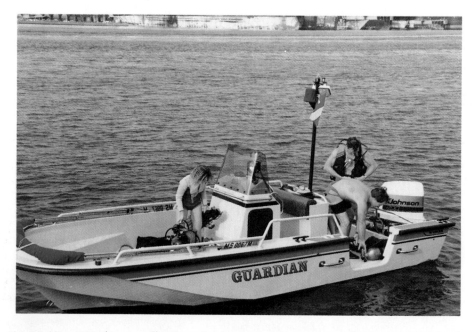

Fig. 5-7 *No matter how small a boat is, there are still certain minimum requirements for equipment safety. (Courtesy of Boston Whaler.)*

and navigation; on larger boats, have someone on board to help. Smaller dive boats that carry six or fewer passengers for hire are required to have only the operator licensed, but the boat is still required to meet certain Coast Guard requirements. If the boat license and operator license are prominently displayed, you can feel more at ease and do less careful checking.

Equipment

Several vital items of equipment are required. There should be more life jackets, more correctly called personal flotation devices (PFDs), than people on the boat. Larger boats need to have a float or raft. Other equipment should include anchors, lines, compass, first aid kit, radio, and oxygen equipment with appropriate regulator and mask for the management of diving accidents. Portable fire extinguishers are required on all boats.

The dive boat should have additional equipment, such as a current line (tag line), extra floats, a recall system, and two types of flags. The red and white sport diver flag should be flown only when divers are actually in the water. It means, "I have a diver down, keep well clear and maintain a slow speed" (Fig. 5-8). The blue and white alpha flag is primarily a boater's flag and means "This vessel has divers below and maneuverability of this vessel is restricted." It is primarily used in international waters and inland navigable waterways when the boat cannot be moved, such as when divers are tethered to the boat by hoses or lines (Fig. 5-9).

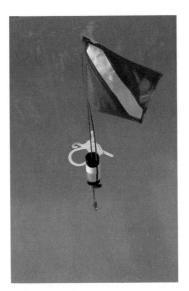

Fig. 5-8 *The sport diver flag warns that divers are in the water.*

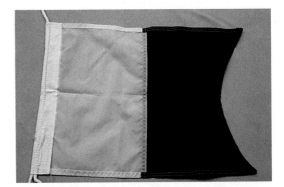

Fig. 5-9 *The alpha flag advises other boats that divers are in the water, that the boat cannot maneuver, and that other craft should stand clear.*

An electronic underwater recall system is used by most larger dive boats. This system sends a warning sound similar to a police siren into the water. The recall system is used when the boat's anchor is dragging, the weather has deteriorated, a diver has an accident, or some other emergency action is needed. If you ever hear such a siren, surface as soon as it is safe to do so and look toward the boat for the crews' signal either to come to the boat or remain where you are.

As boat diving has grown, dive boats have become larger, faster, and more comfortable. Boats used in each diving area may vary in equipment and arrangement. This is based on weather and diving conditions, length of boat runs to dive sites, length of time divers spend on the boat, plus the variety of diving activities done in the area. Some improvements becoming more common include:

1. One or more high-pressure compressors on board
2. Large boarding ramps or platforms and ladders
3. Showers, often with hot water
4. Bunk rooms
5. Galley for food
6. Electronic navigation equipment, including radar, depth sounder, and loran
7. Special dive gear racks

Smaller boats used for shorter trips usually have no room for these items, nor would you need to have them. The smaller dive boats have short runs, usually taking less than an hour to reach a dive site. They usually make only one or two dives per trip with a total trip time averaging between 2 and 6 hours.

Regardless of the size of the boat, make certain that the oxygen equipment on board the boat is in proper working order and that one or more crew members are trained in its use. A quick way to determine whether both of these conditions exist is to ask the captain of the boat to have the crew member designated to handle the oxygen to demonstrate it for you prior to departure. If no one can demonstrate the equipment or if it is inoperable, find yourself another dive boat.

Selecting a Commercial Dive Boat

Once you have an idea of what commercial dive boats look like, how they are equipped, and what you should look for, you will want to actually find a good dive boat. These boats are often chartered by diving businesses or groups. Other times, individual tickets are sold directly. There are several places to find specific information of dive boat trips:

1. Local dive stores
2. Local dive clubs
3. Diving magazines and newsletters
4. Local commercial boat landings
5. National underwater instructor associations
6. Travel agents who specialize in diving trips
7. The yellow pages in harbor areas under "Boats, Charter"

Each of these sources can help you with local boat trips or they may suggest special trips in a diving resort area. Other divers are also good sources of information. Fig.

Boat dive checklist _____

Date(s) of trip: _____

Time of departure: _____   Return: _____

Destination (dive sites): _____

Captain's name: _____

Boat name: _____   Dock location: _____

Directions: _____

_____

_____

Check (√) if the boat has:

Safety equipment _____   Safe entry and exit _____
Oxygen _____   Proper License _____
Galley _____   Sun cover _____
On-board compressor _____   Adequate storage _____

Capacity: _____   Number of divers: _____

Level of diving difficulty: _____

Dive activities: _____

Number of tanks per dive: _____

Location of nearest hyperbaric chamber: _____

Bring own food? _____   Any required sleeping gear? _____

Special local information: _____

Notes: _____

_____

_____

Fig. 5-10 *This is the sort of information you should obtain in planning a boat dive.*

5-10 shows a checklist of questions you need to ask about each dive boat and dive boat trip you are considering.

You may pay for the trip directly to the boat or through the dive store, landing, club, or travel agent. Be sure to take your receipt and/or ticket along with some extra money when you go on a boat trip.

Dive Preparation

You will definitely want to prepare for your trip as thoroughly as possible to ensure a safe and enjoyable boat dive. The first idea is to plan and prepare everything with your regular dive buddy, if possible. You can meet divers on the boat and become buddies for the day, but it is far better to share the entire dive experience with someone you know.

TRAINING AND EXPERIENCE

Unless you learned to dive in an area where boat diving is common, you probably did not receive training for this activity. Some advanced diving courses offer boat diving instruction, if not, ask your instructor to include it in the course.

Diving experience increases your ability to relax and your physical fitness. It maintains skills and teaches you to handle many situations in the water. Diving from shore not only makes you appreciate boat diving more, but also prepares you for this activity. Be sure to select boat diving trips that are within your capability.

Equipment

Particularly when you are preparing for a boat dive, your equipment needs to be at its peak of performance. After all the time of preparation and finally reaching the dive site, plus the cost of the trip, you would not want a piece of equipment to ruin your day of diving. So, pack an extra mask strap, a fin strap, "O" rings, a snorkel holder, a dust cap, a high-pressure plug, wet suit cement, silicone, tape, and so forth. In some cases, the boat crew may have some of these items, but you cannot rely on this, and in some cases their parts may not fit your gear.

Several days before the dive trip, check all your equipment. This gives you time to replace parts, make repairs, and rent replacement gear if something of yours needs to be repaired. Inflate the buoyancy control system, breathe from the regulator, check your tank pressure if you are using your own tank, and carefully go over your wet suit and apply wet suit cement as needed. Check all straps, and so on.

Many dive boat operators provide tanks. If you provide your own, you should have your tank filled, even if the boat has a compressor on board. Boat compressors are often slower and have a lower pressure rating than shore-based compressors and may charge more per fill. By having your tank full, you are ready for the first dive, and if the boat compressor breaks down you can still make this dive.

Your gear should be stored as neatly, securely, and compactly as possible. The tank and weight belt should be kept separate. You either carry them or pass them onto the boat separately while you are loading the boat. One large gear bag for the gear that gets wet and one smaller bag for dry things is a good arrangement. These bags can be either the carry-on or backpack type. Most modern gear bags provide ample space for all your gear, and most divers who do a lot of boat diving carry a plastic bag in their gear bag to keep things dry (Fig. 5-11). Another useful piece of equipment is the dry box, which was shown previously. This is a useful place to store all of your little spare items as well as any small personal belongings that you do not want exposed to water.

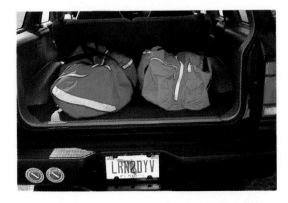

Fig. 5-11 *The gear bag is an essential piece of equipment for boat diving because it enables you to keep your gear organized and in one place.*

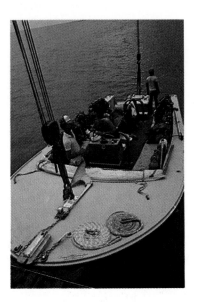

Fig. 5-12 *Underway, the dive gear is stowed, and divers can prepare for the dive or simply relax.*

You will want to pack your gear so that the mask, decompression computer, and other delicate items are separate from each other and are protected by wet suit parts or other soft gear. Before loading your gear bag and after checking each item for proper function, go through the gear in the order you put it on, to make sure you have it all. A list of your equipment is a great help. Then pack gear into the gear bag in reverse order, such as, fins in first and wet suit in near the last so you can put on your gear as you remove it from the bag (Fig. 5-12).

Fitness

You should be generally fit for diving. This includes adequate rest, a well-balanced diet, and regular exercise. Because dive boats often leave during the night or very early in the morning, your sleeping schedule may be disturbed. In addition, you will probably dive more often and deeper than usual on a dive boat trip, requiring you to expend more energy. Therefore, it is important to get as much rest as possible the day or two before the dive and sleep on the boat if possible during the trip to and from the dive site.

The two meals before the boat trip and any food eaten on the boat should be light and nourishing—food you can easily digest. For at least 12 hours before the trip, you should not drink any alcohol and if you use medications other than those prescribed by a physician familiar with diving you should not be diving at all, either on a boat or elsewhere. Another practice to follow for any diving is to make certain that you are adequately hydrated before diving. Dehydration has been found to be one of the factors that may contribute to an increased risk of decompression sickness, so it is important during the 12 to 24 hours prior to any diving to consume substantial amounts of water or other salt-free fluids. The day of your dive trip, any urine that you produce should be clear or nearly clear, indicating that your body is adequately hydrated.

The increased amount of diving done on boats makes it necessary to be able to clear your ears easily. By equalizing the pressure in your ears during the 24 hours before the dive, while on the boat, and at the surface, it is far easier to clear your ears as you descend. If you have difficulty equalizing, you may wish to take some medication. Take only medication you have safely taken before. Bring some of the medication on the trip in case it wears off, do not use medication to mask symptoms that would normally prevent you from diving, and always check with your doctor. These guidelines apply to any other prescription or nonprescription drugs you may need to take; preferably, your physician should be familiar with diving and the effects of diving on certain medications.

DIVE PLANNING

Both you and your buddy should contribute to all dive planning. Above all, you each reserve the right to make the "no-dive" decision, based on changing medical, physical, psychological, or environmental conditions. If something is wrong, do not dive just because you travelled a great distance and paid your money.

Boat diving increases the range of possible diving activities, improves your ability to deal with diving conditions, and makes it possible to come back and regroup if you or your buddy has a problem. Using the dive boat as a surface support station makes the planning and the diving much easier.

Boat Diving Techniques
GENERAL CONDUCT

Boat diving, more than any other diving activity, brings people into close contact. Your behavior affects other divers, just as their behavior affects you. Divers tend to be independent and self-sufficient. This can be balanced and enhanced by the interpersonal relations possible on a dive boat. Each diver should be capable, well-trained, experienced, physically fit, and well-equipped. Still, you can place some reliance on and expect some help from your buddy, other divers, and the boat crew. They, in turn, should be able to expect this from you.

A day of boat diving can be enjoyable and safe if you have a positive attitude and you meet some personal responsibilities. First, look forward to the boat trip, and prepare yourself and your gear. Arrive early, about one-half hour or more before the trip. Ask where you should put your gear and stow it out of the way.

Greet other people while making eye contact and start conversations. Relax and settle down for a pleasant day of diving. This is a good time to find a diving buddy if you do not have one. At this time you will want to find a place to sleep or sit during the boat ride.

Because dive boats are often crowded, it is both a courteous and safer gesture to help someone don a tank, adjust a strap, or adjust a buoyancy compensator (BC). You should keep your gear together as much as possible and work out of your gear bag. As soon as you are back from your dive, put your gear back into your gear bag as soon as you remove it. This keeps the deck neat and prevents the loss or damage of your own equipment. Your gear should be marked with your name or some tape or paint because it is very easy to mix dive gear on a boat. Marking gear also helps tell divers apart underwater.

BOAT PROCEDURES

Look around the boat to get an idea of where things are and get to know the boat as well as possible. Ask the crew or someone who has been on board previously if you need something or do not understand a procedure. These procedures and others have been devised by the boat crew to better serve you. Even if you have been on another dive boat, these procedures may not be obvious. Boats often require you to show your certification card and log book as evidence of currency, and to put your name on a roll sheet and your tank. Some boats supply the tanks and weight belts, and many boats have special ways and places for storing gear.

The marine toilet or head is sometimes quite different from a usual toilet. If instructions are not posted, be sure to ask. Put all trash in the trash can, not in the head, and do not throw any trash overboard. You should stay out of the boat's wheelhouse and engine room. Sometimes the crew may invite you to see the wheelhouse or, if you have a special interest, you might ask to see it. Respect the crew's wishes, as they have a responsibility to all passengers, the boat, and other vessels.

Between dives, relax and take off as much gear as is practical. Most divers leave their wet suits on. Weight belts and tanks in particular should be taken off carefully and as soon as possible. Most boats do not allow dive gear or wet divers in the bunk room or galley. Some boats now allow divers in wet suits to use the galley between dives, but all other gear should still be left outside. The crew can gather items you may need from your bunk. During this time, talk over the interesting sights and events of the dive while planning the next dive. This is also a good time to eat. Be sure to keep your dive gear together and out of the way (Fig. 5-13).

Boats often move to another dive site between dives. This adds to the amount of

Fig. 5-13 When the crew is attempting to find the dive site, it is best not to get in their way.

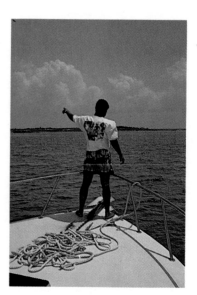

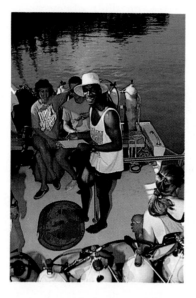

Fig. 5-14 When the divemaster or skipper is taking roll, answer only for yourself.

time you have to relax and prepare for the next dive, as well as providing a surface interval for decompression. During this time the crew fills tanks, or you switch your regulator over to a new tank if there are extra cylinders on board for each diver. Each dive boat has a different system for filling tanks. Some use tags, others have you place the tank in a certain location or remove your pack. If you are using the boat's tanks and they have tank valve covers attached, leave the cover off an exhausted cylinder, since this is usually the way the crew can determine if a tank is empty or full. Be sure you ask your boat crew about the procedure used on their dive boat.

At each new dive site, the crew will tell you the conditions, such as depth, current, special features, and procedures. If you are not clear on a certain point, be sure to ask. Before the boat moves, a visual and verbal roll call is taken. Be sure to answer only for yourself (Fig. 5-14). Some dive boats have a divemaster who checks you in and out of the water for each dive.

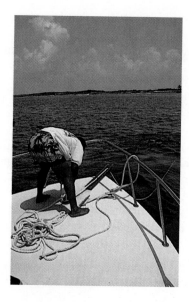

Fig. 5-15 *The mate setting the anchor once the dive site is located. Do not begin to don your gear or enter the water until the skipper gives you the "OK."*

When the crew is handling the anchor, as shown in Fig. 5-15, another smaller boat, or other heavy equipment, stand clear for your own safety. If a diving or boating emergency develops while you are on board, stay out of the crew's way and follow their instructions. Let the crew know if you have special skills, such as medical, mechanical, or instructional that may help.

MOTION SICKNESS

If you have a problem with motion sickness, it is a good idea to eat light, easily digestible foods and take a dose of motion sickness medication 1 to 2 hours prior to boarding the dive boat. Remember to repeat the dosage at the prescribed intervals. Many people feel better if they lie down and sleep. This is aided by many motion sickness medications that make people drowsy. The best place to sleep is down as low and as near the center line and middle of the boat as possible because this part of the boat moves the least. Also, stay away from engine, galley, or head fumes.

Other people can better handle motion sickness by staying on the deck in the fresh air. It is best to watch the horizon because this gives you a steady reference point. If you do vomit, go to the leeward side of the boat near the stern.

PREPARING TO DIVE

Before the first dive, do not rush to get dressed. The skipper often takes time to carefully maneuver the boat right over the dive site and will usually shut off the engines. Be sure the skipper gives the "OK" before you get ready or enter the water.

As you put on your dive gear, help your buddy and let your buddy help you. Hold the tank as your buddy puts it on and then reverse the process. Do not put a tank on over your head because there is the possibility of hitting someone, or falling if the boat moves. Never leave your tank standing unattended, because it could be knocked over very easily. Be careful to lean forward and step into your weight belt and not swing it around you. This avoids hitting some other diver. You should also avoid sitting on the deck when other divers are donning gear, since your head is right at the level of other divers' tank bottoms.

When you and your buddy are dressed, do a complete buddy gear check (Fig. 5-16) and review your dive plan away from the boat's exit/entry point to avoid congestion. Put your fins on last, near the exit point so you will not need to walk in them.

Depending on how the dive boat is arranged and the number of divers on board, you may need to jump into the water from some height (Fig. 5-17). It is not

Fig. 5-16 *Check your buddy's gear thoroughly prior to the dive.*

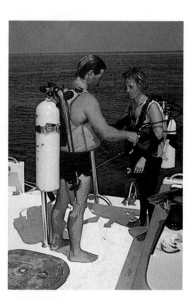

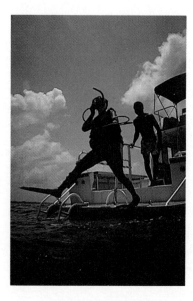

Fig. 5-17 *On some boats, the giant stride will be the preferred form of entry.*

always necessary for you to jump; you may be able to climb down a ladder or roll off the ramp or swim step, or simply perform a seated entry if the seas are not too rough and an appropriate dive platform is available on the boat (Figs. 5-18, 5-19, 5-20). When you jump into the water, as shown in Fig. 5-17, you should use the following procedure in performing the giant stride:

1. Use the lowest exit point.
2. Put some air into your BC.
3. Put your mask in place and your regulator in your mouth.
4. Secure your octopus and weight belt.

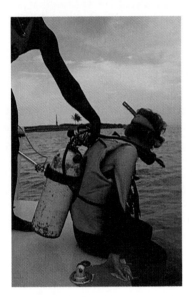

Fig. 5-18 *The controlled seated entry, if seas are calm enough, is the easiest way to exit the dive boat.*

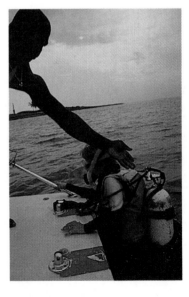

Fig. 5-19 *The diver slips carefully into the water from the platform.*

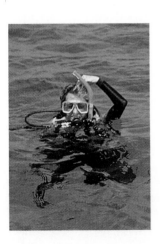

Fig. 5-20 *As soon as you are in the water and secure, turn and face the boat and give the "OK" sign.*

5. Watch the swing of the boat and be prepared to enter the water as the boat is swinging away from your intended point of entry.
6. Look to see that the water is clear.
7. Hold your mask and regulator with one hand and look out at the horizon.
8. Step off the boat or dive platform in the giant stride.
9. Turn and signal to the divemaster that you are "OK" before descending.
10. When there is wind, stay away from the sides of the boat, particularly when diving in kelp.

Once you are in the water, have any accessory gear, such as cameras, handed down to you. A line of 8 to 12 feet with a clip is good for this when seas are rough. Then, move away from the boat on the surface and look back to the boat and wait for your buddy. Before descending, do one more buddy check.

THE DIVE

One of the many advantages of boat diving is that you can often descend and ascend right by the boat, eliminating the need to snorkel. After your final buddy check on the surface, clear your ears, even though you have not yet started to descend. Go on scuba, if not already using it, deflate your BC, hold your inflator/deflator hose above your head, exhale, and begin your descent. It is best to descend slowly and feet-first, while controlling your buoyancy, clearing your ears, checking your instruments, and keeping track of your buddy. A slow descent can be assured by properly weighting yourself and not over-weighting. You can use the anchor line or a descent line for descending or ascending, but if the boat is rising and falling in a surge, keep the line at arm's length.

Be aware of currents by observing seaweeds, bubbles, or your drift. If there is a current, swim into it on your dive so you can return with the current at the end of the dive. In areas of very strong currents, nearly all diving is done from boats. One method of current diving is to anchor the boat and dive in an area up-current from the boat (Fig. 5-21). A line called a lead line is attached from the anchor line, directly to the stern of the boat. Another line with a float, called either a current, trail, or tag line, is trailed to the stern. You enter the water holding the lead line and pull yourself to the anchor line and then on down. You do not kick when you are on the line. At the bottom, you dive into the current and then return by the anchor line, to the lead line, then to the stern of the boat, and out of the water.

A float dive in a current is done with a float on the surface and a line to the divers on the bottom (Fig. 5-22). As the divers move, the boat follows the float. At the end of the dive, the divers surface by the float and are picked up by the boat. Drift diving is done by picking up the boat's anchor off the bottom and letting the boat drift with the divers. You stay near or hold onto the anchor line as you drift (Fig. 5-23).

Another form of drift diving, often called live boating, is usually done from larger dive boats. In this case, the boat is underway, clear of divers, and does not have any anchor or floats in the water. You and your buddy get completely ready and enter the water as close together as possible. You should know the compass

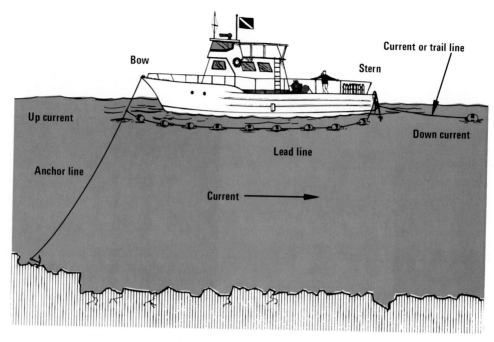

Fig. 5-21 *The line arrangement above is used for current diving with the dive boat at anchor.*

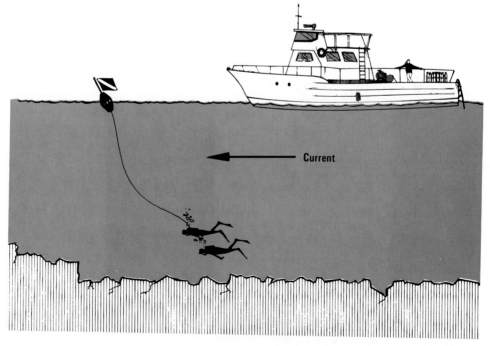

Fig. 5-22 *Float diving is another method for diving with a current.*

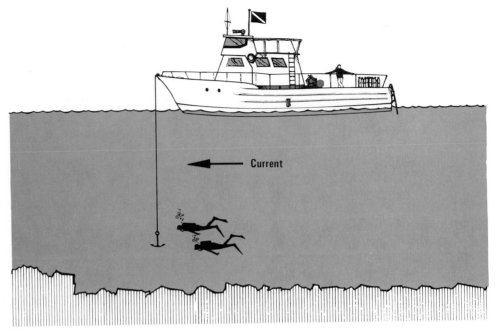

Fig. 5-23 *A drift dive is another approach to diving in a current.*

course of the drift so you later know where to look for the boat. You and your buddy make the dive drifting free with the current. At the end of the dive, surface very carefully—looking up, raising one hand, moving slowly, and listening.

On the surface, you and your buddy fully inflate your BC and join any other divers who are nearby. The boat usually starts down-current, picking up divers, so you are drifting toward the boat (Fig. 5-24). Wait for the boat to come to you while you get ready. When the boat arrives, listen and watch for the crew's instructions. Be sure to do what they say. When the boat stops with the props out of gear, or you are given the "come on" signal, board as quickly as possible with all your gear in place.

When you dive in currents, just as in deep diving, wreck diving, and night diving, go with a diver who is experienced in this type of diving. Preferably this would be an instructor or divemaster.

If your dive is quite far from the boat's anchor, it is common practice to surface after you have used one-half to two-thirds of your air and check the boat's position. This presumes your dive does not require decompression stops. Some divers like to do this several times during the dive. Each time you surface during a dive, give the surface "OK" sign to the crew so they will know you are not having a problem but simply checking your location.

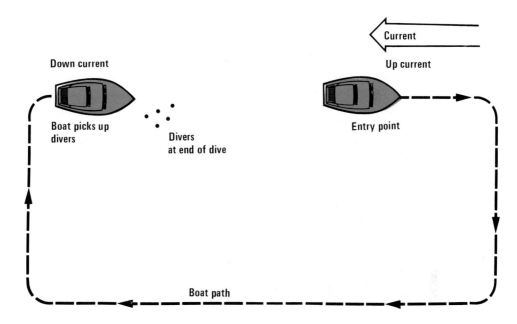

Fig. 5-24 *Live boating drops the divers into the water and the boat then comes to the proposed end of the dive route and picks up the divers from down current.*

Each successive dive of the day should be shallower than the previous dive; on each successive dive, stay closer to the boat and make your activities less strenuous. Your diving will be safer and more enjoyable this way. If water conditions permit, go skin diving instead of scuba diving on the last dive. Remember, you are diving to relax and enjoy yourself. This is far more important than what you find or how much of the bottom you cover.

Returning to the Boat

When you and your buddy agree to return to the boat, you may want to surface swim if you are low on air. Inflate the BC to raise your body well out of the water. If you have plenty of air, you can take a compass bearing and return underwater. As mentioned above, give the "OK" sign to the boat as soon as you are on the surface, regardless of which return method you plan to employ. Also, if seas are really rough, you will find going easier underwater. If you plan to stay on the surface while returning to the boat in rough seas, be sure to have adequate air, keep the regulator in your mouth, and continue to breathe from your tank.

In returning to the boat by means of a compass underwater, remember that the boat is a smaller target than the shore, so you need to be more careful when doing return navigation underwater. Adjust for any drift as you swim and allow for any swing of the boat around its anchor. If the boat is swinging when you take your bearing, set your course for a point between the bow and where you imagine the anchor to be resting.

Watch for any natural aids to navigation, such as rocks, weeds, wreckage, and so forth, that you passed on the way out. Also, listen for the boat's compressor or generator so you will know when you are getting close. If you swim longer than expected, surface and adjust the course. Do not swim just under the surface of the water because other boats cannot see you; instead, control your buoyancy and swim 10 to 20 feet underwater, along the bottom, or in mid-water if visibility is good.

Any ascent should be done with your buddy at a very slow, easy pace, while using the BC to reduce the work of swimming (Figs. 5-25 and 5-26). To assure proper ascent rate, allow air to leave the BC as you approach the surface and the "bubble" expands in volume. Be sure to look up, hold your hand up, go slowly, pause between 10 and 20 feet for 3 to 5 minutes, listen for other boats, and then proceed to the surface.

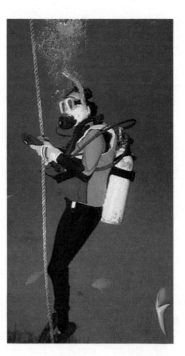

Fig. 5-25 Ascending the anchor line, the diver must still monitor ascent rate.

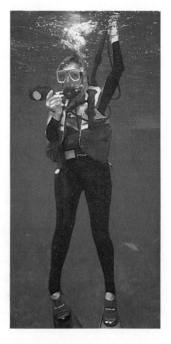

Fig. 5-26 While performing a free ascent, the diver must monitor the ascent rate and watch for overhead obstructions.

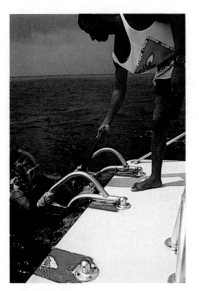

Fig. 5-27 *The weight belt is first handed up to the divemaster, and if the seas are calm enough the fins may be handed up as well.*

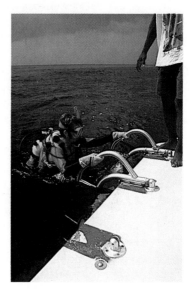

Fig. 5-28 *The diver begins to exit the water. Note that the diver still has the regulator in her mouth. She will exit the water with all equipment still in place.*

If you arrive at the boat's anchor line or you have surfaced up the boat's anchor line, it is often easier to swim underwater beneath the boat directly from the anchor line to the ladder, ramp, or dive platform at the stern. Surface slightly behind and to the side of the stern to observe the wave and boat action. Be sure the area is clear before you move in and then come in with your head well above the water and take secure hold of the ladder, ramp, or platform, keeping it at arm's length. Remove your weight belt first and hand it up to the crew member tending the exit point (Fig. 5-27). Next, hand up any accessory gear that you may have had on your dive, such as a camera. Depending upon wave conditions, you may wish to hand up your fins before reboarding the boat. In calm seas, you can safely hand your fins to a crew member since swimming without them should the boat swing slightly should not be too arduous without the fins. However, in rough seas, the fins should be kept on your feet while getting back on board the boat. This will give you strong swimming ability should you lose your balance reboarding the boat after a dive (Fig. 5-28). If many divers are attempting to get back on the boat at the same time, stay clear of the exit point and hang onto the tag line. This will prevent you from becoming injured by a falling diver or tank, in the event one of the divers ahead of you should slip and fall backward while getting back onto the boat. Another safety precaution has to do with the dive platform or ladder in rough or choppy conditions: Pay special attention to the boat and platform as it pitches. Do not get caught under it as it falls.

If you should surface down-current from the boat, you will have the current against you as you swim back. There are several choices to ease this situation:

1. Swim to the tag (current) line, if it is closer than the boat, and pull yourself in, hand-over-hand, being careful not to become entangled in the line. Be sure to watch the boat as you pull yourself in
2. Swim underwater on the bottom, using a compass course
3. Swim on the surface with the BC inflated
4. Signal by hand or whistle for help from the boat
5. Swim across the current to a nearby shore, hike up-current beyond the boat and then drift or swim back to the boat
6. Swimming on your back may be easier and less exhausting.

If you should miss the boat during drift diving, the current line is available so you can pull yourself back in. Most swimming methods already mentioned are not useful in strong currents of 2 to 8 knots. If you miss the line, inflate your BC and wait for the boat to pick you up.

There is a remote chance that you might be left or missed by the dive boat or your own boat may drift away. This could happen from the anchor dragging, a boating or diving emergency causing the boat to move, or an inaccurate roll call. If this happens, be calm and stay with your buddy. You will be missed and a search will begin.

If you are near shore when the boat misses you, swim in and get out of the water. If you are far from land, get maximum positive buoyancy. As time passes, ditch any gear that is a hindrance; however, keep your mask, snorkel, fins, BC, and wet suit. Stay together and in the area unless you know exactly which direction to swim to decrease the time it takes for the boat to find you.

Post-Dive

As soon as your dive is over, pack your gear away. It is easier to pack your gear when the boat is not moving. If the boat has a shower, just wash yourself, not your gear, with a quick shower, because boats have a limited supply of water. The trip back is a perfect time to sunbathe, sleep, talk, eat, or drink. Be sure you know the procedure for paying for any food, drinks, or air on the trip back. Before you leave the boat, be sure you have all your dive gear and personal belongings.

Just as the anticipation and planning for a dive is as much a part of diving as the dive itself, so is the sharing of your diving experience. Of course, you and your buddy will have the most in common to share, but all divers will have similar experiences to relate. If you have made your dives with a positive and open-minded attitude, even a difficult day with rough or dirty water can be satisfying and you can gain in your diving experience. If you enjoyed your trip let the deck crew and divemasters know. If they were helpful and courteous, tipping may be appropriate. The crew of most charter boat operations depend on tips to supplement their base wages. These energetic people put in long days, often arriving hours before you do and staying to clean up long after you are gone. Tips always improve their spirits following a long dive day, in addition to making your return trips that much better. One way or another, they will remember you the second time around.

Boating for the Owner-Operator

Boating and diving have a great deal in common. Both are demanding, yet rewarding activities and an effective blend of them can increase your recreational pleasure. Training, proper equipment, skill, experience, and planning are vital in boating and diving; communications, rescue, first aid, weather, and navigation are also common to both activities.

U.S. COAST GUARD REQUIREMENTS

The Coast Guard does not require private boats or the operators of private boats to be licensed unless they are carrying passengers for hire. It is important to remember that fines can be very heavy if you carry passengers for hire without the proper license. Certain equipment and other actions are required by the Coast Guard and other governmental agencies. The nature and number of these required items vary with the size and type of boat. The categories include:

1. Boat registration and numbering
2. Accident reporting
3. Rules of the road
4. Boat ventilation
5. Pollution control
6. Personal flotation devices
7. Fire extinguishers
8. Back-fire flame arresters
9. Signalling equipment
10. Navigation lights
11. Oxygen equipment

Equipment

If you own a boat and use it for diving, there is some additional equipment you should consider carrying. What you actually decide to carry depends on the size of the boat, the area of operation, and the type of diving activities. Remember, diving equipment can also be used to solve boating problems, such as untangling a propeller or anchor or searching for equipment lost overboard.

Boating safety and first aid equipment includes:

- First aid kit and book
- Oxygen with high-flow delivery capability
- Fire extinguishers

- Personal flotation devices
- Signal equipment
- Flares
- Bailing or pumping equipment
- Blankets

Diving operation and support equipment includes:

- Current (tag) line and float
- Extra floats
- Diving flags (sport diver flag and alpha flag)
- Extra scuba unit and weights
- Lines for tying off gear and for safety stops
- Extra mask, snorkel, and fins
- Dive tables
- Diving textbook
- Diving emergency information
- Book of local dive site information

Boat operation and support equipment includes:

- Radio
- Compass
- Anchors and lines
- Ladder
- Tie-down lines
- Engine spare parts
- Tools
- Extra lines
- Boating publications and charts
- Knife
- Boat hook
- Flashlight
- Depth sounder

Comfort and convenience equipment includes:

- Trash container
- Motion sickness medication
- Towels and rags
- Water

SELECTING A BOAT

Because of the tremendous variables in boats and diving, it is not possible to provide a complete review of boat selection. But if you want your own diving boat, some general ideas will help you (Fig. 5-29).

Dive from a commercial dive boat in the area you intend to use your boat. Carefully observe how the boat is equipped, handled, and which dive sites are used; go

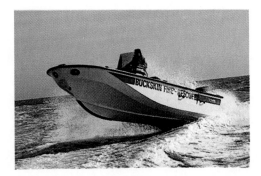

Fig. 5-29 *Small boat suitable for scuba. (Courtesy of Boston Whaler.)*

boating with a friend or rent a boat and try boating in the area; and take a course in boating from either the U.S. Coast Guard Auxiliary or the U.S. Power Squadron. These courses are very low in cost and a great introduction to small boats and safe small boat handling. You might also visit several local boat dealers and look over the more popular boats sold in the area.

Be aware that a private boat intended for diving should have an easy way to enter and exit the water. Some newer boats feature a water-line entry feature that makes entering the water and returning to the boat quite easy. The boat should be durable and not fancy because tanks and weights are hard on boats, and it should have room for both dive gear and boat equipment. Make sure the boat is suitable for local weather and water conditions and is capable of carrying more weight than you intend to put in it. Any boat you choose should also adapt to other activities, such as water skiing, fishing, cruising, and the like.

Having your own boat is a significant investment of your effort, time, and money. With this investment comes additional responsibilities to your passengers and other boaters. You may decide that for the investment, you are better off diving from commercial boats. But, if you decide that having a boat is best for you, you should be strongly committed to this combination of boating and diving. Learn all you can about these skills so you can become adept at both.

Small Boat Techniques

Whether you are using your own boat or a rental boat, there are certain techniques that are most appropriate for dive trips taken in small boats:

1. Advise someone who is not going of your boating plan, including time of return.
2. Check the weather report.
3. Keep both dive gear and number of divers to a safe, comfortable number.
4. Organize all dive equipment for ease of access in a minimum of space.
5. Check out another person on the boat in case something happens to you. This includes using the radio, starting the engine, hoisting the anchor, maneuvering the boat, and locating and using the emergency equipment on board.

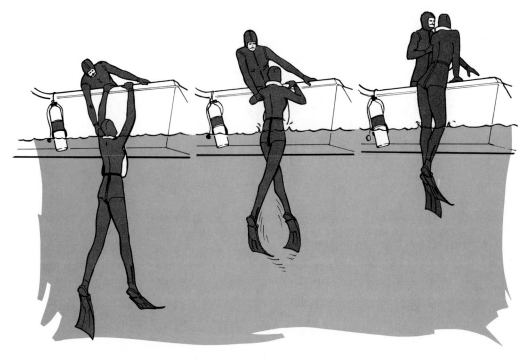

Fig. 5-30 *The steps in reentering the small boat. Notice that gear has been removed.*

6. Secure loose gear while underway.
7. If the boat is very small and the trip is short, you might suit up on shore.
8. If you put on gear while in the boat, stay low, move slowly, and be careful.
9. Anchor as near as possible to the dive site and stay out of any traffic or hazardous areas. If moorings are used in your area, *do not anchor*, use the moorings.
10. Be sure the anchor or line secured to the mooring is secure before the dive and, if anchored, check the anchor when you reach the bottom.
11. Leave a qualified person on the boat, if possible.
12. Fly the red-and-white sport diver flag only when people are actually diving, and fly the alpha flag as well.
13. If you are in a current area, put out a current line with a float.
14. Keep track of weather and sea conditions and seek shelter at the first sign of bad weather.

The back-roll is a good entry from a small boat. If the boat is very small, this should be done simultaneously by two divers on opposite sides of the boat. Provide a sturdy ladder to climb out of the water or a line to tie off gear to aid in boat entries. When entering a small boat with no ladder, place accessory gear, such as cameras, spears, and other equipment, carefully in the boat or tie them off. Then remove your weight belt, tank, mask, and snorkel and place them in the boat one item at a time. You may want to tie off your weight belt and tank. If you are wearing a BC that has considerable bladder volume in the front, you may want to deflate the BC before trying to enter the boat. To actually enter the boat, hold the gunwale, and give a strong kick with your fins while hoisting yourself up with your arms (Fig. 5-30). Let your buddy help you and you in turn should help your buddy.

When you make a beach landing in a small boat, watch the sets of waves for some time outside the surf line. During this time, you can be strapping down equipment and checking to see that you have enough fuel. The best time to go through the surf is immediately after a big set of waves because waves that follow will be at lower levels. This gives you time to unload and remove the motor before the next cycle of big waves.

The support and added convenience of a boat can make your boat diving experiences some of your most memorable. This is especially true if you keep safety uppermost in your mind by using proper etiquette on board and correct techniques in the water.

6 *Underwater Navigation*

OBJECTIVES

At the conclusion of this chapter you should be able to:

1. Explain the difference between latitude and longitude.

2. Name several sources that may be consulted to obtain navigational charts.

3. Describe the various types of compass that may be used in diving and the relative merits of each.

4. Explain the meaning of variation and differentiate it from deviation.

5. Name the three components that must maintain a proper relationship in order for you to follow a compass course exactly.

6. Explain how to compute a reciprocal compass course.

7. Describe how to take current into consideration when determining an underwater compass course.

8. Tell how you can determine the amount of distance travelled underwater so that you can accurately follow an underwater compass course.

9. Name the three simple rules that should be followed in order to increase your chances of success during a search and rescue effort.

10. Determine what is the most important factor to consider when selecting an underwater search pattern.

KEY TERMS

Parallels	Meridians	Sailing charts
General charts	Coastal charts	Harbor charts
Small craft charts	Compass card	Variation
Magnetic north pole	True north pole	Deviation
Lubber line	Course line	True course
Magnetic course	Magnetic heading	Reciprocal course
Compass Rose		

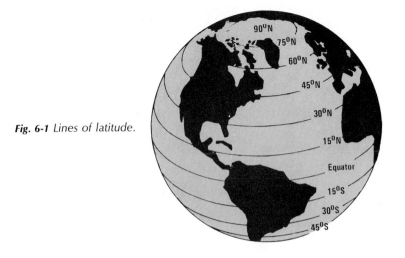

Fig. 6-1 Lines of latitude.

Navigation had become an exacting science long before the first scuba equipped diver broke the bonds from diving bells and air hoses, to freely explore the mysteries of the deep; it was not long before the time-honored principles of seafaring navigators were applied to underwater navigation.

Navigating at depth is quite simple, in fact, most of what you need to know you have probably already experienced. Distances are the same as those on the surface, time does not change, and directions are identical to those with which you are already acquainted. The only difference is that you also have the third dimension—depth. Your diving experience is enhanced when you know where you are going and, more importantly, how to get back. You will find that a basic understanding of the tools of navigation and how to properly use and interpret them instills confidence in your diving abilities.

This chapter introduces a variety of navigation aids, such as charts, the function and use of the compass, and how to plot and swim a course under various conditions. Correctly applying these skills lets you utilize your bottom time to the utmost and dive longer with safety by conserving your air and energy.

The Earth

Any serious study of navigation must eventually begin with the earth. Past navigators designed a grid system of latitude and longitude that surrounds the earth and forms the basics by which position is determined.

The ends of the earth's rotational axis define the geographic North and South poles. Halfway between the poles is an imaginary line, called the equator, which divides the earth into the Northern and Southern hemispheres. The equator is the starting, or zero degree, point of latitude. Fig. 6-1 illustrates that lines of latitude,

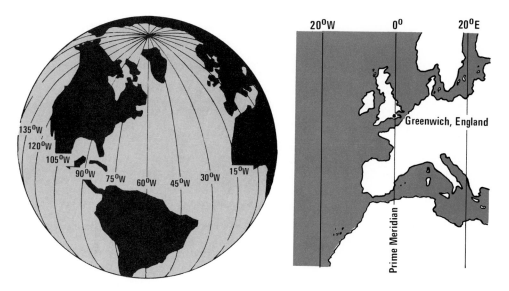

Fig. 6-2 *Lines of longitude.*

or *parallels*, are evenly spaced north and south of the equator and are labelled in degrees. The poles are 90 degrees north and south.

Lines of longitude, or *meridians*, make up the east and west references of the grid system. Through international agreement, the zero-degree longitude line, called the *prime meridian*, was established as a line running from the North and South Poles through the old Royal Observatory in Greenwich, England. From the prime meridian, the globe is divided into 180 degrees in each direction to establish the Eastern and Western hemispheres, as shown in Fig. 6-2. Early mapmakers used this simple grid system to chart the globe. Today, this system is used to accurately pinpoint positions or intended destinations on navigation charts.

Navigation Charts

Charts are nothing more than a diver's road map. When properly used, charts open a whole new world of diving adventure. Charts provide detailed information about the depth of water in fathoms, shorelines, topographic features both above and below the surface, aids to navigation, dangers, and other information of interest to both navigators and divers.

There is a variety of charts available. It is important to understand the differences between each and select the chart most appropriate for your needs. There are four basic navigation charts of interest to divers: sailing, general, coastal, and harbor or small craft charts. Each chart, and for that matter, charts of the same type, differ in scale. Scale is the ratio of a given distance on the chart to the actual distance it represents on the earth.

Sailing charts vary in scale from 1:1,200,000 to 1:600,000. This means that 1

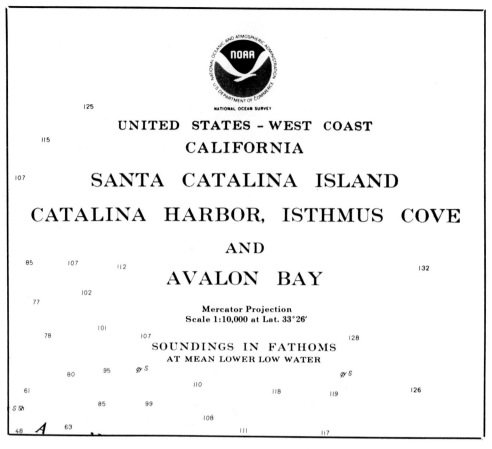

Fig. 6-3 Harbor chart.

inch equals between 16 and 8 nautical miles, respectively. They are used primarily for long-range seafaring navigation and provide a general overall view of certain areas. Detail is minimized and only the major topographic features are represented.

General charts range in scale between 1:600,000 and 1:100,000; 1 inch equals approximately 8 to 1 nautical miles, respectively. They are used to plot courses along the coast and to give boaters a slightly more detailed view of a particular area.

Coastal charts range down to a scale of 1:50,000, where 1 inch on the chart equals a little more than half a nautical mile. As the name implies, the charts primarily show outlying reefs, shoals, and bays or harbors of considerable width.

The charts listed so far are primarily used by the boater and are not of much value for a diver working along the shore. However, *harbor charts* or *small craft charts,* as shown in Fig. 6-3, have a scale from 1:50,000 down to 1:5000, or a range from one-half mile down to where 1 inch equals only 139 yards. These charts depict great detail and provide the information you need to locate specific objects or diving areas.

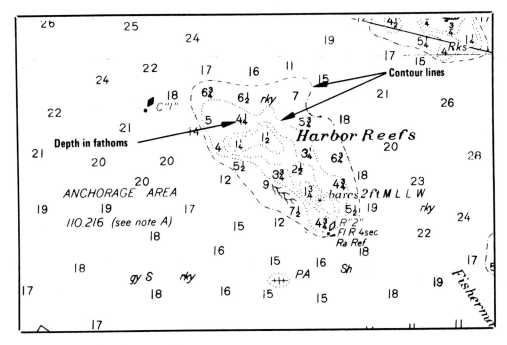

Fig. 6-4 *Depth and contour lines.*

CHART SOURCES

Several government agencies publish and sell navigation charts. The most common charts are put out by the National Oceanic and Atmospheric Administration (NOAA), the National Ocean Survey (NOS), the Defense Mapping Agencies Hydrographics Center, and the United States Lake Survey Center. Most dive stores, marine stores, and some Government Printing Office bookstores have catalogs available to help you select the appropriate chart.

CHART SYMBOLS

Chart information is portrayed by a set of standard symbols and color codes. To gain the maximum benefit from the chart you select, you should become familiar with its symbology. Depth, for example, is marked in either feet or fathoms. A fathom, as you recall, is 6 feet. Contour lines, shown in Fig. 6-4, connect points of the same relative depth. In addition, the depths above 30 feet are color-coded within each zone so you can instantly recognize them. This gives you a good indication of the relative depth of any dive.

Chart symbols are also used to point out submerged and partially submerged objects and their actual depths (Fig. 6-5). Charts show rocks and reefs, and which ones are covered and uncovered at both high and low tide. Furthermore, they indicate the type of bottom and its quality within any given area. Charts also depict reference points or landmarks that help you locate or relocate exciting dive spots.

Partially submerged wreck	Rock	Landmark	Quality of Bottom	
↙	⊛	⊛ *Eagle Rk (rep 1955)*	*G*	*Gravel*
			Sn	*Shingle*
			P	*Pebbles*
			St	*Stones*
			Rk; rky	*Rock; Rocky*
			Blds	*Boulders*
			Ck	*Chalk*

Fig. 6-5 *Chart symbols.*

The margins of the chart contain the degrees of latitude and longitude. Each degree is divided into 60 equal units, called *minutes*, and each minute is further subdivided into 60 *seconds*, as shown in Fig. 6-6. One minute of latitude represents 1 nautical mile, or about 6076 feet. Determining latitude and longitude enables you to pinpoint exact locations on the chart and either relay that information to others or record the precise location of an object.

Correct use of these underwater charts can greatly enhance your diving experience, not only for locating items, but also for the enjoyment of studying the charts and preparing for other exciting dives.

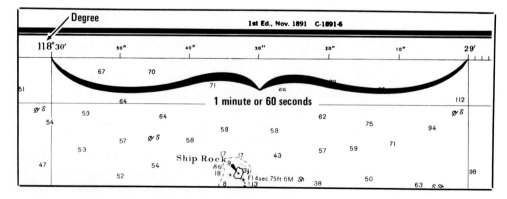

Fig. 6-6 *Degrees of longitude.*

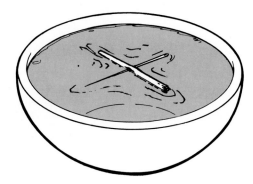

Fig. 6-7 *Early compass.*

Compass

The key instrument to underwater navigation is the compass. To some people, the compass is a mysterious and magical instrument. The truth is that the compass is not only a simple device, but it is also an essential, basic safety tool.

The main purpose of a compass is to aid in directional control. To you this means the ability to relocate offshore dive sites or return to the shore or boat, without having to surface to orient yourself. A compass is particularly valuable when surface conditions are less than ideal. Wave action, adverse surface currents, and boat traffic make surfacing away from your intended exit point potentially dangerous. The compass becomes as valuable as any other piece of life support equipment carried by the safety conscious diver.

When combined with charts, the compass can help you more easily locate underwater reefs and known shipwrecks and add more time for pleasurable exploration to each dive.

COMPASS PARTS

To understand compass function, you must first understand the parts of a compass. The original compass was nothing more than an iron needle that a ship's pilot rubbed against a lode stone. The lode stone was a chunk of magnetized iron ore with the ability to magnetize other bits of the same metal. The magnetized needle was pushed through a piece of straw and floated in a bowl of water, as shown in Fig. 6-7. The magnetic attraction of the needle made it point toward the Magnetic North Pole.

Today's more sophisticated compass is much more reliable and accurate than its early predecessor. It is still, however, a relatively simple tool. Compasses come in a wide variety of shapes, sizes, and types.

A magnetic needle suspended in a liquid-filled encapsulated housing is one type of compass. This compass has an outer ring or bezel depicting the degrees of a circle and may be fixed in place or rotating. A lubber's line indicates the line of position and parallels the centerline of your body. The compass has removable straps so that it may be placed on the wrist, mounted on a compass board, or placed in a console.

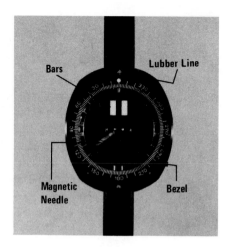

Fig. 6-8 Top-reading navigation compass.

The familiar top-reading compass is shown in Fig. 6-8. This compass has a fixed outer ring, or bezel, depicting the degrees of a circle. The lubber's line has an arrowhead at the north or zero degree position on the bezel. Two large bars can rotate to align with the desired course on the bezel. To maintain the selected course, you keep the magnetic needle between the bars and sight along the lubber's line.

TYPES OF UNDERWATER COMPASSES

Several considerations must be kept in mind when selecting a compass, such as how you intend to use it, the product's quality, how well it functions, and, of course, how much it costs. The general categories of compasses are the watchband, the wrist-mounted top- and side-reading, and the more sophisticated compass boards used primarily for competitive navigation courses (Figs. 6-9 through 6-12).

The first thing to determine when selecting a compass is how you intend to use it. If you want one for general directional control to return to your point of entry, a

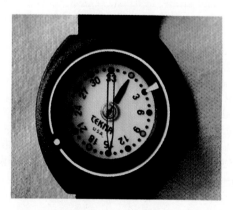

Fig. 6-9 Watchband compass.

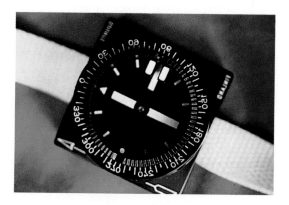

Fig. 6-10 *Top-reading navigation compass.*

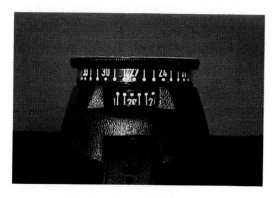

Fig. 6-11 *Side-reading wrist compass.*

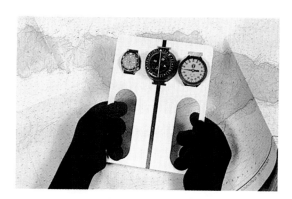

Fig. 6-12 *Board-mounted compass.*

simple, durable compass may be sufficient. On the other hand, if you need a compass capable of precise navigation, like the ones required in commercial diving or competitive compass runs, you may want the board-mounted compass. For the vast majority of divers who want dependable, reasonably priced compasses that are easy to use, one of the top- or side-reading compasses is certainly the most desirable and practical.

Watchband Compass

The watchband compass, shown in Fig. 6-9, provides general directional information that enables you to return to a predetermined area with a fair degree of accuracy. This type depicts only the cardinal points of a compass and should not be used for navigation in poor visibility or where a high degree of accuracy is required.

A positive aspect to the watchband compass is its small size. It is always attached to the watch and can be referred to at any moment without worrying about an additional compass or remembering to put it on or take it off. These compasses are very durable, require almost no maintenance, and with merely reasonable protection from extremely hard use, last a long time. Watchband compasses are also inexpensive.

Top-Reading Compass

The top-reading, or mariner's compass, as shown in Fig. 6-10, comes in a wide variety of qualities. Your demands on the compass should determine the quality of the compass you buy. Styles range from a very inexpensive compass with minimal quality and dependability to the more sophisticated compasses commonly found on boats.

A good top-reading diver's compass should have, as minimum requirements, degrees around the outside, on the bezel, marked on the compass body itself, or on a floating compass card. It should have a movable bezel, which enables you to set a predetermined course and reciprocal, or reverse, course under readily visible points. The compass should be sensitive, but not so sensitive as to react to every metallic item along the course. The compass also should not have a significant lag or slow response. It needs to respond quickly enough so any off-course deviation is immediately noted. The compass should also have a strap or some means of securely attaching it to your body; at the same time, it should be easy to remove in case you want to hold it for a more accurate navigation procedure.

Side-Reading Compass

The side-reading, or aviation, compass, as shown in Fig. 6-11, is essentially the same as the top-reading compass, both in style and quality. The only difference is that it provides directional information that can be read from the side. It is also designed primarily to let you hold the compass in your hand or on your wrist in front of your face to maintain a visual line of sight while reading the compass.

Board-Mounted Compass

The final type of compass used in diving is the board-mounted compass, as shown in Fig. 6-12. This compass is used exclusively for precision navigation, such as that required in competitive navigation courses or for the commercial or military diver who must locate exactly a specific spot or return via some complex route.

A board-mounted compass can be either a side- or top-reading compass. These compasses are, however, of a quality generally found either on boats or airplanes and are used for cross-country navigation or cross-water navigation where extreme dependability and accuracy are absolute requirements. Generally, they are very expensive and range in design from a simple solid-mounted, liquid-filled compass to a compass mounted on a base that stays level at all times and responds instantly to the slightest course deviation.

COMPASS CARE AND HANDLING

After a dive, the compass should be washed, cleaned, and relubricated. Remove all sand, dirt, and saltwater deposits from the case. Relubricating, in most cases, means nothing more than simply spraying the compass with silicone after a thorough washing. Full attention should be given to the bezel to make sure it moves freely enough so you can adjust it underwater with gloves on, but with enough resistance so it will stay in place once you have set it.

Compasses, by their very nature, tend to be a bit fragile and therefore, like cameras or watches, require careful handling. If your compass is to maintain its quality and dependability, the magnetic needle has to move freely. When transporting any compass, pack it carefully inside your gear bag to protect it from damage, as shown in Fig. 6-13. Pack and handle a board-mounted compass very carefully so it will not be thrown off the settings. Given this kind of care, your compass should last a long time and give you good, accurate, dependable service.

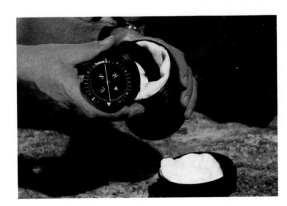

Fig. 6-13 *Packing the compass.*

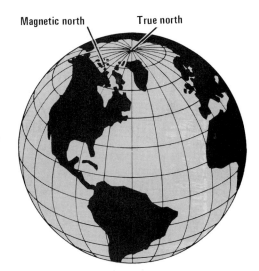

Fig. 6-14 *Magnetic north.*

VARIATION

A basic consideration with a compass is that it point to the *Magnetic North Pole,* which is approximately 1000 miles south of the *True North Pole,* as shown in Fig. 6-14. Therefore, when the compass points to 0 degrees or magnetic north, it is not necessarily pointing to true north. Variation is the difference, expressed in degrees, between true north and magnetic north.

There are points within the United States where there is no variation between magnetic north and true north. This is when the True and Magnetic North Poles are in line. A line drawn through these points is called the *agonic* line (Fig. 6-15). The compass will read 0 degrees and there will be 0 degrees variation. But points either east or west will have a variation, depending on how far west or east they actually are. Variation is designated as east or west on all charts, depending on whether the magnetic needle is deflected to the east or west of true north. To convert the course you draw on a chart to a magnetic course that you can follow with a compass, apply this popular saying: "east is least and west is best." This means you should subtract easterly variation and add westerly variation.

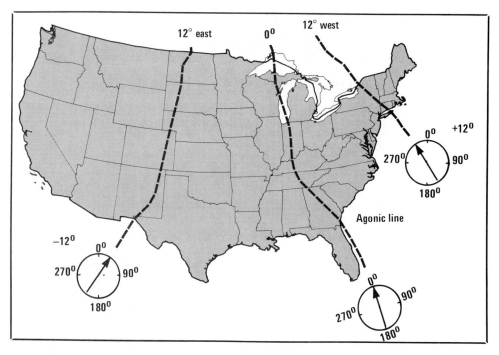

Fig. 6-15 *Magnetic variation.*

Two methods are commonly used for portraying variation. On small-scale charts where large distances are shown in small areas, lines that connect points of equal variation are drawn. On large-scale charts, such as those most often used by divers, a compass rose is used (Fig. 6-16). The outer compass rose is oriented to true north, while the inner compass rose points to magnetic north. The difference between the two is the variation. The degrees of variation are also labelled in the middle of the compass rose.

Variation changes only slightly from year-to-year by the shifting of the earth's molten core. The change each year is calculated and noted on nautical charts.

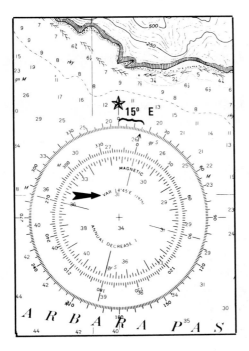

Fig. 6-16 *Compass rose.*

DEVIATION

Another common inherent compass error is *deviation*. Deviation is created by the magnetic interference of metallic objects within the immediate vicinity of the compass and the inherent error of the compass itself. On a boat it could be something as simple as a metal can or set of keys near the compass. While diving, deviation can occur when the compass is held too close to metallic objects worn by you or your buddy such as tanks or cameras. For this reason, you should be aware of metallic objects around you or on your person that might create deviation. Metallic objects you pass over on the bottom could also create deviation.

Generally, you have very little control over magnetic interferences caused by metal objects on the bottom. You do, however, have control over the interference of metal objects you wear. To determine how your equipment affects your compass, arrange the equipment on the ground and move the compass around it. You can determine which equipment has the greatest influence on the compass and the best position to hold the compass to minimize the effects of deviation.

On the surface, deviation can be accepted to a large extent because the compass generally is not relied on exclusively for directional control. You can go from one sighted point to another sighted point, or along a course where there are other objects on which you can take a heading, sometimes called a sighting, fix, or bearing. However, underwater it is sometimes impractical, if not impossible, to rely on visual sighting to maintain a course. For this reason, greater reliance on the compass

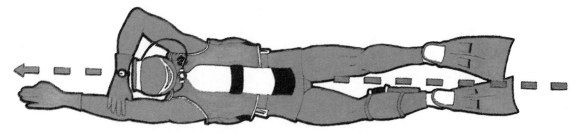

Fig. 6-17 *Using the compass.*

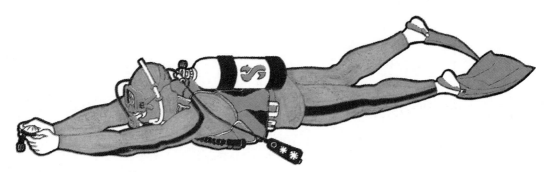

Fig. 6-18 *Holding the compass.*

is essential. Be continually on guard for deviation influence by observing the surrounding terrain within your range of vision. You should be able to determine if you are moving in a straight line or moving at some angle to the intended source.

TIPS ON USING THE COMPASS

To use a compass underwater, take the hand that has the compass and grasp the opposite arm at the elbow. Your opposite arm should be pointing in the direction you plan to swim (Fig. 6-17). This technique provides a solid base for the compass and aligns the lubber's line or direction-of-travel arrows with the centerline of your body. This allows you to more easily follow the compass heading. Hold the compass level. When tilted too far, the compass card will no longer move freely and will drag on the compass body, preventing accurate direction control. A problem with this technique is that it quite often places the compass in immediate proximity to the mask, tank, and in some cases, other gauges. To minimize deviation, avoid as many metallic objects as possible.

For more precise navigation, you may find it desirable to loosen the compass from the wrist and hold it out in front of you with both hands, as shown in Fig. 6-18. This technique provides the same solidarity as the armlock method and moves the compass far enough away from metallic items that can induce magnetic deviation.

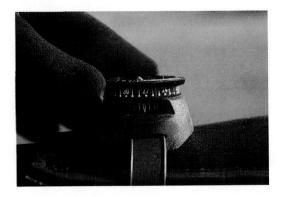

Fig. 6-19 Navigating with side-reading compass.

Fig. 6-20 Navigating with top-reading compass.

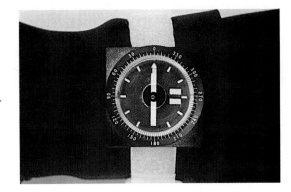

The compass is commonly installed in an instrument console that houses other gauges and related instrumentation such as depth gauge, submersible pressure gauge, and decompression computer. Care must be taken to minimize the likelihood of deviation caused by the close proximity of metallic objects.

If you are to navigate underwater accurately, the compass course must be followed exactly. This means maintaining a relationship between the compass, lubber's line, and body. For example, assume you have the type of compass depicted in Fig. 6-19 and you want to swim a westerly course of 270 degrees. Hold the compass with the lubber's line exactly parallel to the length of your body and move until 270 degrees, or west, is directly behind the lubber's line. Maintain this relationship as you swim and you will follow a 270 degree heading.

If you have the type of compass shown in Fig. 6-20, and you want to swim the same westerly course, set the movable bracket lines on the face of the compass opposite 270 degrees on the bezel. Then move until the compass needle is between the brackets. To maintain the heading, simply keep the compass needle between the bracket lines and sight along the lubber's line. When the correct position has been established, you should think of your direction of travel as a line passing directly through your body, intersecting the compass lubber's line and pointing precisely to your destination.

Once you understand these key relationships and have mastered a simple out course and then reciprocal courses you are ready for the more advanced underwater navigation techniques. These techniques can include such things as triangular courses and the more complicated techniques as used for surface navigators.

Using Charts and Compass Together

Select a chart for the diving area of your preference. The easiest procedure when using a chart is to always turn the "north" of the chart toward true north. Then, when you draw your course line on the chart, it will be pointed in the actual direction you intend to swim.

Next, draw a line with a straightedge from your starting point to your destination. This is your *course line* (Fig. 6-21). After you draw the line, one method you may use to navigate is to select objects along the course line, such as reefs, wrecks, shelves, buoys tied to the bottom, or other objects, and plan to swim from one object to the other. It makes no difference if they are slightly off the desired course, you can still reach you destination. This technique of using objects for checkpoints is desirable even when you swim a course by compass, because it lets you continuously monitor your progress and helps you more easily maintain the course.

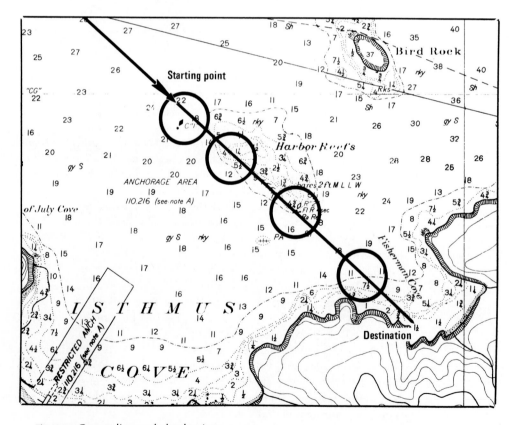

Fig. 6-21 *Course line and checkpoints.*

The other method is to accurately measure the course as an angle from true north. To do this, you need a protractor, marine plotter, or an air navigation plotter, similar to the one shown in Fig. 6-22. Align the baseline of the plotter with the course line. Then, with the center of the plotter over a line of longitude, read the *true course* from the plotter rose (Fig. 6-23). (Small arrows are printed on the rose to indicate the scale to be used for your direction of travel.) Double-check your answer by mentally visualizing the general direction of the course.

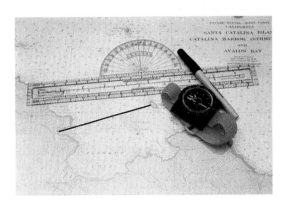

Fig. 6-22 *Navigation plotter.*

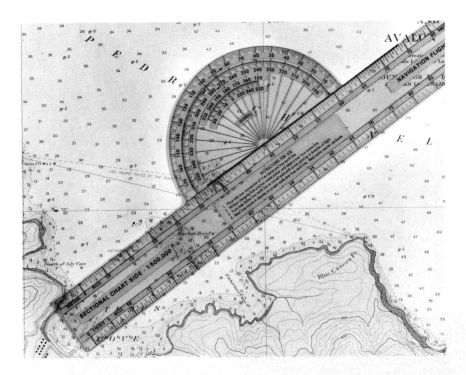

Fig. 6-23 *Measuring true course.*

At times, the course line may not cross a line of longitude. To determine the true course, simply extend the course line until it intersects a line of longitude. Then use the procedure just described to find the true course.

Next, add or subtract the magnetic variation for the area. The amount of variation is obtained by reading the value from the nearest variation line or the compass rose nearest your course line. (You may have to interpolate for your position on the chart.) The value you have after subtracting or adding variation is called the *magnetic course*. If you do not have to compensate for currents or tide, this value is the heading you set on your compass. It is called the *magnetic heading*.

Reciprocal Dive Courses

Before you can compute a reciprocal dive course (in which you come back on the same course line you followed going out) you must first determine the compass heading for the outbound course. For example, assume the outbound course is 290 degrees (west/northwest). The return, reciprocal, or inbound course is 180 degrees from the outbound course. In this case, it would be 110 degrees (290 degrees − 180 degrees = 110 degrees), or east/southeast. Because the outbound course is 290 degrees, it is easiest to subtract 180 degrees. If the outbound course is less then 180 degrees, the proper procedure would be to add 180 degrees. By predetermining these figures and setting the compass on 290 degrees, you can follow the compass heading out and enjoy the dive. To return to the boat, set the compass on 110 degrees and follow it back. The more computations you can do before the dive, the more you will enjoy the dive.

Advanced Navigation
CURRENTS

When you dive, you become part of your environment and are affected by its movement. This means that as the water moves, you move, or drift with it. For example, if you maintain a northerly heading while diving in a 1-knot (1 nautical mile per hour) current from the east, you will drift with the current, or westward (Fig. 6-24). In fact, after 1 hour, you will be 1 nautical mile to the west of your intended course. To compensate, you must turn *into* the current to a heading that will let the current drift you along the desired course line.

To dive in waters with current you must know two additional factors: the speed and direction of the current and your underwater swimming speed. Tidal current tables and tidal current charts are available from the National Ocean Service. Through their use and actual observations, you can estimate possible current speed and direction.

To determine your swimming speed, swim a predetermined course over the bottom and either count the number of kicks to establish a feet-per-kick speed, or time the course and determine your feet-per-minute speed. The latter of the two is the most accurate for navigational purposes. The course should be repeated several times to achieve an accurate swim rate.

To determine the compass heading that compensates for the current, use a sim-

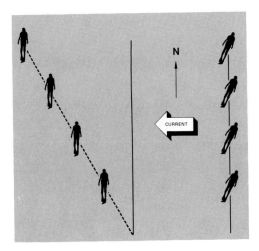

Fig. 6-24 Drift correction.

ple vector diagram, or a diagram that shows course or compass direction. You can draw this diagram on the navigation chart or on a separate piece of paper. The important item is to establish a true north line.

The first step is to plot and measure the true course. As shown in Fig. 6-25, the true course from point A to point B is 300 degrees. The direction and speed of the current is plotted next. Always use the same unit of measure to plot speeds.

The current, as read from the tidal current tables, is toward 45 degrees and the speed is 1 knot. To make the speed easier to plot, 1 nautical mile per hour is converted to 2 feet per second (6076 feet ÷ 3600 seconds = 1.69 feet per second, rounded to 2). From point A, the current line is drawn in the direction of the flow. The length of this line to point C is the speed of the current, 2 feet per second (Fig. 6-25).

The next item to enter is your own swim speed, which we will assume to be 180 feet per minute. The value is converted to 3 feet per second (180 feet ÷ 60 seconds = 3 feet per second). The same scale on the plotter is used to plot the swim speed. You may use either scale as long as it is the same one you used to measure the length of the current line, and you continue to use the same scale for all measure-

Fig. 6-25 True course, current direction, and speed.

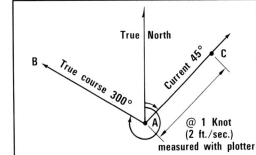

ments. Place 3 over point C and move the zero mark on the plotter until it intercepts the true course line (A, B), as shown in Fig. 6-26.

The angle formed by the true north line and the swim speed line (C, D), is the true heading for the dive, 260 degrees (Fig. 6-27). The drift correction angle is 40 degrees left, into the current (C, D, A). Variation is then applied to this heading to achieve the compass heading for the dive.

The length of the line from point A to point D is the speed over the bottom you will maintain under these conditions. In this case, it is 1.8, which is rounded to 2 feet per second (Fig. 6-27). This speed is used to calculate how long it will take you to swim to your destination. In this example, assume the distance from A to B is 600 feet. Use the basic formula (distance ÷ speed = time) to compute the swim time. The distance, 600 feet, is divided by the speed over the bottom, 2 feet per second, to find the swim time of 300 seconds or about 5 minutes.

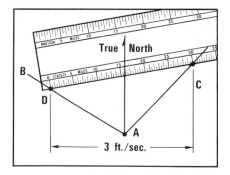

Fig. 6-26 *Plotting swim rate.*

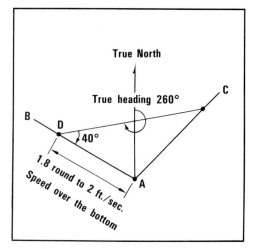

Fig. 6-27 *True heading and over-the-bottom speed.*

Reciprocal Courses in Currents

When you have computed your compass heading to your destination in a current, simply planing the return on a reciprocal heading will put you considerably off course. The correction you held *into* the current on the way out must be matched by a correction into the current on the way back.

The reciprocal course must be computed from the true course and correction angle applied to it, but in the opposite direction. In the previous example, the true course was 300 degrees. The reciprocal course, therefore, will be 120 degrees (300 degrees − 180 degrees = 120 degrees). The correction angle was 40 degrees left to compensate for the 1-knot current from the left. Since the current will be from the right on the return trip, it is added to 120 degrees. The true heading for the return trip is 160 degrees. Again, variation must be applied to arrive at a compass heading for the return dive.

MULTIPLE COURSES

Once you feel comfortable with computing navigation courses, reciprocals, and current problems, the next step is to work with routes that follow more than two headings. In a triangular course, you follow three different headings to return to the original point of departure (Fig. 6-28). Another navigation problem you may encounter is one in which you have two groups of divers who are following separate courses and who want to meet at a predetermined point (Fig. 6-29).

Each dive requiring navigation skills is computed using the same basic navigation techniques described earlier. Once a specific course has been plotted, the compass headings and swim times are computed separately for each leg. With more than one course to follow, it is helpful to write each compass heading and swim time on your slate for quick reference.

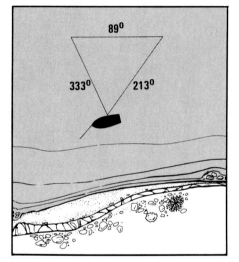

Fig. 6-28 *Triangular course.*

Fig. 6-29 *Multiple course dive.*

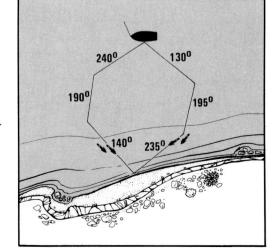

SEARCH AND RECOVERY

This specialty type of diving requires a great deal of skill, accuracy, training, and coordination. If you are not experienced or are unfamiliar with the techniques used in search and recovery, it is not a good idea to try it. As a general rule, you must be an excellent navigator, both at the surface and below; be able to coordinate search patterns, regardless of the number of divers or the visibility; and be thoroughly familiar with the techniques of safely rigging and raising objects of all sizes to the surface.

An understanding of *simple* search and recovery techniques can help you find a piece of equipment that has accidentally gone overboard. Leave heavy search and recoveries to the professionals.

Your odds of success are increased if you follow three simple rules: define the search area, select the best search pattern, and establish a system of keeping track

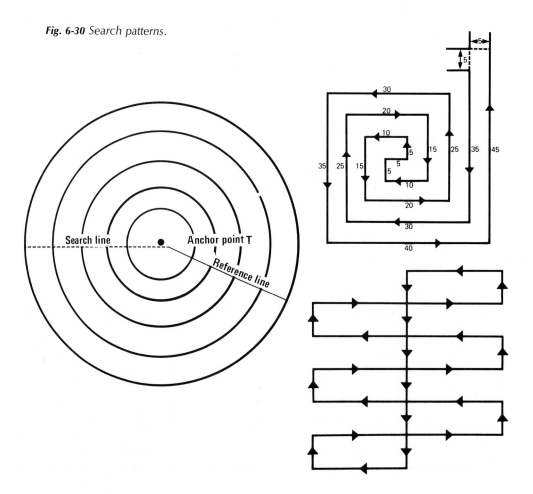

Fig. 6-30 *Search patterns.*

of the areas that have already been searched. Bearing or coordinates can be used to define the basic search area and where to anchor. Currents or tidal movement are sometimes factors that should be considered.

The search pattern you select depends, to a large part, on the number of divers involved and environmental conditions. It could be a simple compass course or an elaborate gang sweep of the area (Fig. 6-30). The important factor is to keep it as simple as possible. Once a certain area is searched, have a system for checking it off. This eliminates excessive overlap and duplication.

When you have located an object that is too large for you to retrieve alone, mark its location. Buoys are the best method for marking location. You will most likely have spent a lot of time and effort to locate the object and surfacing before the location is marked means you may have to spend as much time relocating it.

Applying Navigation Skills

To see the practical application of using charts and compasses, let us follow a typical buddy team from the time they are at home planning a weekend dive through the actual dive. With charts scattered from one end of the living room to the other, they evaluate the places they have been and the places they might go, and try to decide where to dive this weekend. Eventually, they come across a chart of Santa Catalina Island and a harbor chart of Isthmus Cove on Catalina (Fig. 6-31). They decide that this is the place, since they know of a previously lost anchor and two other intriguing areas near Bird Rock in this area.

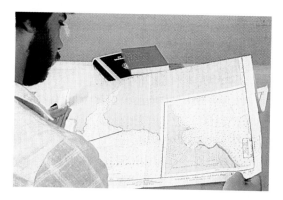

Fig. 6-31 *Santa Catalina and Isthmus Cove.*

PREDIVE PLANNING

When they arrive at the Isthmus, they plot their dive plan on the chart for future reference and begin the actual preparation for the dive. Using a harbor chart, they first plot the true course from the Isthmus landing to a spot 50 yards northwest of Bird Rock where they plan to anchor (Fig. 6-32). They find the true course to be 40 degrees, north/northeast. The variation, as indicated on the charts, is 14 degrees

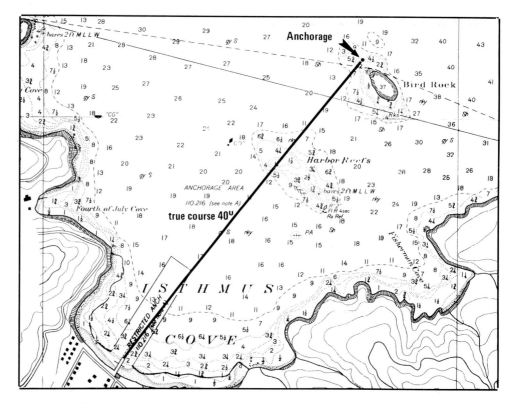

Fig. 6-32 *True course to anchorage.*

45′ east, which is rounded off to 15 degrees (Fig. 6-33). Subtracting this from the true course gives a compass heading of 025 degrees. The chart also indicates a depth of 12 feet at the planned anchorage. They load their gear into the boat and head to the dive site.

Once anchored, they begin the predive checklist, using their diving log. First, they make note of the actual location of the anchorage near Bird Rock. The true course from the Isthmus was 040 degrees, and by taking a bearing from the rocks on the northwest corner of Bird Rock, they determine the exact location to be 33°27′6″N, 117°29′14″W. The distance from the Isthmus landing is approximately 1520 yards (Fig. 6-34). They also note the conditions at the anchorage. The weather is beautiful and sunny, the water is calm, there is no current, and they have more than 100-foot visibility with a water temperature of 70° F and an air temperature of 85° F.

They now begin to plot their actual dive courses. The first destination will be the mound or rise on the bottom just north of Bird Rock (Fig. 6-35). The true course is 040 degrees, which was the same as the course from the Isthmus landing. Since they do not have to compensate for current, they simply subtract the variation of 15 degrees east and arrive at a compass heading of 035 degrees. The distance to the mound is computed to be 100 yards. They each have previously determined

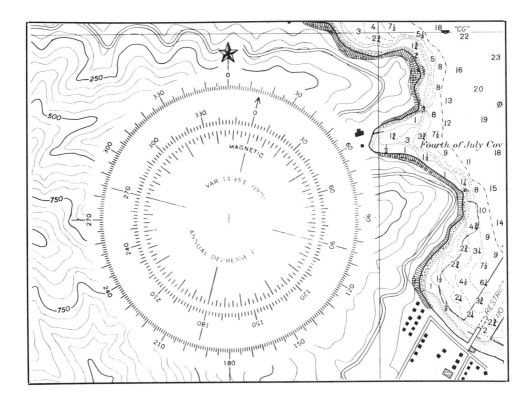

Fig. 6-33 *Magnetic variation compass rose.*

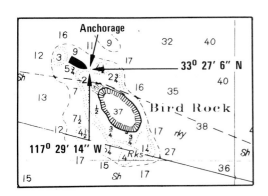

Fig. 6-34 *Anchorage location.*

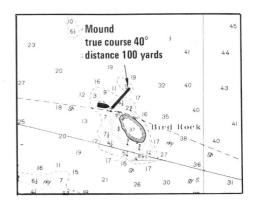

Fig. 6-35 *Course to the mound.*

their swim rate to be 60 feet per minute. With the distance and swim rate known, they are able to estimate the time required to reach the mound. After converting the swim rate to 20 yards per minute (60 feet per minute; 3 feet = 20 yards per minute), they compute that it will take 5 minutes to swim 100 yards (100 yards; 20 yards per minute = 5 minutes).

The next step is to find how much air they will use to reach the mound. The depth of the mound is 9 fathoms, which converts to 54 feet. They estimate that the average depth during the dive will be 30 feet and their surface air consumption rate is 25 psi per minute. Referring to the air consumption tables, they note that with a surface consumption rate of 25 psi per minute, their air consumption rate at 30 feet will be 47.5 psi per minute. For 5 minutes, they will use 237.5 psi. The information for this leg is entered in the dive log.

On the second leg of the dive, they will try to locate the lost anchor. They estimate its position and draw the true course (Fig. 6-36). The anchor should be 100 yards south/southeast of the mound on a true course of 162 degrees. The magnetic heading will be 147 degrees. At a swim rate of 20 yards per minute, it will take 5 minutes to reach the anchor. The planned average depth for this leg is again 30 feet and the air consumption is calculated to be 237.5 psi. This information is written on the dive log.

The third leg of the dive will be the return trip to the boat (Fig. 6-37). From the estimated location of the lost anchor to the boat, the true course is 281 degrees and the magnetic heading is 266 degrees. The distance is 100 yards and, again, it will take 5 minutes to complete this. Due to the rapidly rising terrain on the return

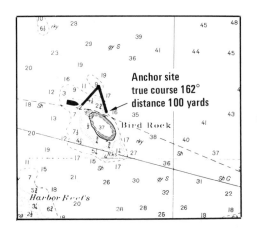

Fig. 6-36 Course to anchor site.

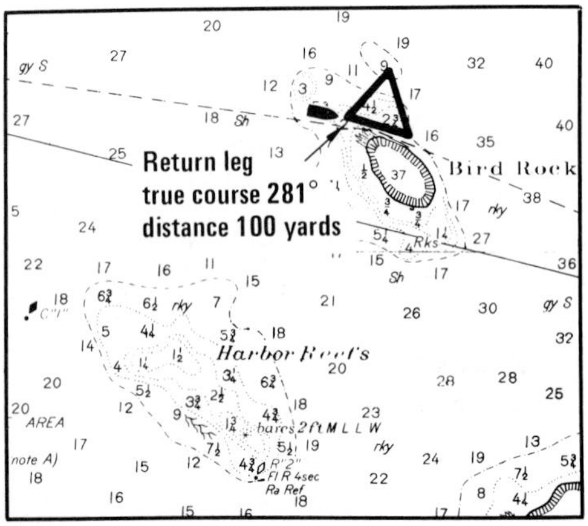

Fig. 6-37 Return course.

trip, they estimate their average depth to be 15 feet. From the air consumption table, they determine the air consumption rate at 36.3 psi per minute. For the last leg, they will use 181.5 psi.

With the course planning complete, as shown in Fig. 6-38, the divers now determine how much time they will be able to spend at each destination based on the total air volume of their tanks and predetermined dive plan. Each diver has 3000 psi of air. The air consumed on each leg is added for a total of 656.5 psi. They also want to return to the boat with a reserve of at least one-third of their total air supply, which is 1000 psi. This is added to the air consumed during the swim for a total of 1656.5 psi. This figure is subtracted from the total air pressure of the tank, which leaves a total of 1343.5 psi of air to be divided between the mound and looking for the anchor.

ISTHMUS LANDING TO ANCHORAGE
True Course - 40°
Compass Heading - 25°
Distance - 1,520 Yards

LEG·1 TO MOUND
True Course - 40°
Compass Heading - 25°
Distance - 100 Yards
Dive Time - 5 Minutes
Average Depth - 30 Feet
Air Consumed - 237.5 p.s.i.
Time at the Mound.

LEG·2 TO THE ANCHOR
True Course - 162°
Compass Heading - 147°
Distance - 100 Yards
Dive Time - 5 Minutes
Average Depth - 30 Feet
Air Consumed - 237.5 p.s.i.
Time at the Anchor.

LEG·3 RETURN TO THE BOAT
True Course - 281°
Compass Heading - 266°
Distance - 100 Yards
Dive Time - 5 Minutes
Average Depth - 15 Feet
Air Consumed - 181.5 p.s.i.

Fig. 6-38 *Course planning.*

Both divers agree that they would like to spend as much time as possible at both sites and that looking for the anchor may take a little longer. Therefore, they decide to spend 10 minutes at the mound and 13 minutes looking for the anchor.

With the top of the mound at a depth of 54 feet, they assume that most of their time will be spent at around 60 feet. Their air consumption rate at 60 feet is 70 psi per minute. For a 10-minute dive at this depth, they will consume 700 psi. The average depth in the area of the lost anchor is 30 feet and, at this depth, their air consumption rate is 47.5 psi per minute. The total consumed in 13 minutes will be 617.5 psi. The total air consumed at both dive sites is 1317.5 psi, which is well within the total air available. They recheck all of their calculations (Fig. 6-39).

DIVE CALCULATION

LEG I TO MOUND
TRUE COURSE - 40°
VARIATION - 15° E
CURRENT - 0
DISTANCE - 100 YDS.
AVG. DEPTH - 30 FT.
SURFACE AIR CONSUMPTION RATE -
25 PSI PER MIN.
SWIM RATE - 60 FT. PER MIN.

COMPASS HEADING = TC 40° - 15° EV = 25°
TIME TO MOUND =
1. CONVERT 60 F.P.M. TO YDS. PER MIN. =
60÷3 = 20 YDS. PER MIN.
2. DISTANCE 100 YDS. ÷ 20 YPM = 5 MINUTES
AIR CONSUMED -
1. FROM AIR CONSUMPTION TABLES, CONSUMPTION RATE AT DEPTH OF 30 FT. FOR A SURFACE CONSUMPTION RATE OF 25 PSI PER MIN. IS 47.5 PSI PER MIN.
5 MIN × 47.5 PSI PER MIN = 237.5 PSI

LEG II TO ANCHOR
TRUE COURSE - 162°
VARIATION - 15° E
CURRENT - 0
DISTANCE - 100 YDS.
AVG. DEPTH - 30 FT.
SURFACE AIR CONSUMPTION RATE -
25 PSI PER MIN.
SWIM RATE - 60 FT. PER MIN.

COMPASS HEADING = TC 162° - 15° EV = 147°.
TIME TO ANCHOR = (SAME CALCULATION AS LEG I)
AIR CONSUMED = (SAME CALCULATION AS LEG I)

LEG III RETURN TO BOAT
TRUE COURSE - 281°
VARIATION - 15° E
CURRENT - 0
DISTANCE - 100 YDS.
AVG. DEPTH - 15 FT.
SURFACE AIR CONSUMPTION RATE -
25 PSI PER MIN.
SWIM RATE - 60 FT. PER MIN.

COMPASS HEADING = TC 281° - 15° EV = 266°.
TIME TO BOAT =
1. CONVERT 60 F.P.M. TO YDS. PER MIN.
60 FPM ÷ 3 = 20 YDS. PER MIN.
2. DISTANCE 100 YDS. ÷ 20 YDS PER MIN. = 5 MIN.
AIR CONSUMED =
1. FROM AIR CONSUMPTION TABLES, CONSUMPTION RATE AT DEPTH OF 15 FT. FOR A SURFACE CONSUMPTION RATE OF 25 PSI PER MIN. IS 36.3 PSI PER MIN.
5 MIN. × 36.3 PSI PER MIN. = 181.5 PSI

TOTAL AIR CONSUMED FOR 3 LEGS =
237.5 PSI
237.6 PSI
181.5 PSI
SUB TOTAL 656.5 PSI
PLUS RESERVE + 1000.0
1656.5 PSI

TOTAL IN TANKS 3000.0 PSI
- 1656.5 PSI
1343.5 PSI REMAINING TO USE AT MOUND AND LOST ANCHOR SITE.

• MOUND -
10 MIN. AT AVG. DEPTH OF 60 FT. WITH A CONSUMPTION RATE OF 70 PSI PER MIN. =70 PSI PER MIN. × 10 MIN. = 700 PSI PER MIN.
• LOST ANCHOR -
13 MIN. AT AVG. DEPTH OF 30 FT. WITH A AIR CONSUMPTION RATE OF 47.5 PSI PER MIN. = 47.5 PSI PER MIN. × 13 MIN. = 617.5 PSI

617.5 PSI + 700 PSI = 1317.5 PSI.
1343.5 PSI REMAINING AIR
- 1317.5 PSI PROJECTED USE
26.0 PSI SURPLUS TO ADD TO RESERVE

Fig. 6-39 Rechecking calculations.

The Dive

Having detailed the dive plan and gained familiarity with each other's equipment, the divers finish their predive checklist. They dress and check each other for correct equipment assembly and adjustment. As shown in Fig. 6-40, they note in their logs the size of their tanks (80 cubic feet) and their starting psi (exactly 3000 psi for each of them).

DATE_____

DIVE LOCATION: _CATALINA ISLAND, ISTHMUS, BIRD ROCK_____

DIRECTIONS: _1520 YDS. 40° NNE FROM ISTHMUS LANDING_____

COORDINATES: _____

CONDITIONS:

WEATHER	SURFACE	CURRENT	VISIBILITY	
☑ Sunny	☑ Calm	☑ None	☑ Excellent	WATER TEMPERATURE _70°_
☐ Cloudy	☐ Choppy	☐ Light	☐ Good	
☐ Overcast	☐ Rough	☐ Medium	☐ Poor	AIR TEMPERATURE _85°_
☐ Stormy	☐ Stormy	☐ Heavy	☐ None	

DIVE BUDDY(S) _RON BLAKE_____

PRE-DIVE CHECK LIST

BUDDY GEAR CHECK	SAFETY PROCEDURE	TIME IN:		(YOU)	(BUDDY)
☑ Adjustment	☑ Depth	_10:05_	Tank Size	_72_	_72_
☑ Buckle Location	☑ Minimum PSI Prior to Surfacing (500)				
☑ Octopus	☑ Direction 25° NNE, 147° SSE	TIME OUT:	PSI Start	_3,000_	_3,000_
☑ Air On	☑ Compass Heading 266° NNW				
	☑ Lost Buddy Procedure	_____	PSI Return _____		

REPETITIVE DIVE CALCULATIONS

Depth	Bottom Time	Repetitive Group	Surface Time	New Depth	New Group	No Decomp Time

WITNESS: _____

DIVE NARRATIVE (use back for complete details)

Fig. 6-40 *Dive log.*

The divers note the time (10:05) and then enter the water and swim the 025 degrees magnetic heading to the mound. Five minutes later, they arrive at the top of the mound, check the depth gauges, and note that they are at 54 feet (Fig. 6-41). They move down to a maximum of 60 feet where they take some pictures. At exactly 10:20, they start for the area of the lost anchor along a magnetic heading of 147 degrees.

When they arrive at the anchor site 5 minutes later, they start a circular search pattern. The anchor is located in a few minutes and they tie it to an inflatable buoy to mark the location so they can retrieve it on a second dive. They finish their 13 minutes by taking more photographs of some lobsters (Fig. 6-42).

At 10:38, they reset their compasses to 266 degrees and head back to the boat. After 5 minutes, they find themselves directly under the boat. Because there is no current, and the dive has been particularly restful, they find they have 1250 psi left in their tanks. So, they decide to continue their dive under the boat until they have reached either the limit of allowable bottom time of their predetermined air termi-

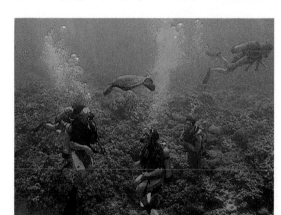

Fig. 6-41 The mound.

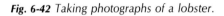

Fig. 6-42 Taking photographs of a lobster.

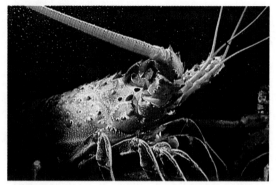

nation point, at which time they will surface. Their plan must accommodate for air and time required to complete any safety stops on their return to the surface.

Upon surfacing and removing their gear, they fill in their log sheets and prepare for any repetitive dives. They note their psi on return is 500 psi for the first buddy and 600 psi for the second buddy. They complete their dive profile and, after a rest, they move back to pick up the anchor knowing precisely what their repetitive dive schedule should be.

By following this procedure, the divers are able to complete their dive safely, fulfilling their objectives. They were able to go directly to each dive site, spend their allotted time, and return well within predetermined safety limits. They achieved their purpose on the dive, and prevented any undue or excess exertion. They were able to enjoy the dive itself, along with the anticipation of the dive through predive planning.

Planning each dive can add a whole new dimension to your diving skills. It can help eliminate a "hit or miss" dive, increase familiarity with underwater terrain, help relocate good dive sites and, best of all, add that extra something that makes a dive more than "just for fun."

Once these skills have been mastered, you are availed of an entirely new activity in recreational diving. You can use charts to locate new and exciting diving spots. You can move to and from any predetermined location, based on simple navigational techniques, without the necessity of surfacing to reorient. Diving in general becomes safer and more fun, and it gives you a new sense of capability. Navigation also opens up a potentially new area of the sport for competition. The basics are simple and enjoyable and all they require is practice.

7 Limited Visibility and Night Diving

At the conclusion of this chapter you should be able to:

1. Explain how to use a diving light when diving in turbid water.

2. Describe several natural direction finders that may be utilized when diving in limited visibility situations.

3. Explain how to control ascent and descent rates and the use of a diving light for monitoring rates of ascent and descent.

4. Tell what should be taken into consideration when using the compass in limited visibility situations in salt and fresh water, with deviation in mind.

5. Tell the cardinal rules when diving with a buddy in a limited visibility situation.

6. Describe how bioluminescence occurs.

7. Explain that relative to water clarity, what should be a key safety consideration when night diving.

8. Name the piece of equipment that can be utilized for communication should you and your buddy become separated on the surface.

9. Describe the various types of light that are available for night diving and the relative features of each.

10. Name the one diving activity that is particularly suited to night diving.

KEY TERMS

Thermoclines	Upwelling	Tunnel vision
Vertigo	Nocturnal	Chemical glow lights

One of the most important environmental factors affecting diving activities is underwater visibility. It can range from over 300 feet to zero. Specific examples of visibility are a range of 75 to 150 feet in the Bahamas and an average of less than 30 feet in the Great Lakes.

To dive safely in limited visibility, there are certain special considerations. You need to know what makes water "dirty" and how to recognize it. Before entering this type of water, you must have the correct equipment and a thorough dive plan.

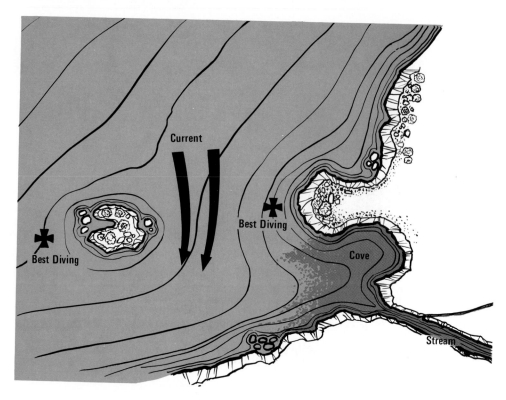

Fig. 7-1 *Best diving during runoff.*

Once you are in the water, your knowledge and training will help you use the right procedures for limited visibility diving. Your procedures must be tighter, your plans better, and your senses keener than when diving in clear water. Night diving is in a class by itself, although you use similar techniques for both diving in turbid water and at night. Predive planning and safety requirements are especially important for a successful night dive. A calm attitude is essential for limited visibility diving, but if you are equal to the challenge it offers, the rewards are high.

Turbid Water

To experience both the pleasures and problems of turbid water, it is necessary to understand what turbid water really is. Low visibility water is referred to as "turbid" because it not only contains dirt, but also has a variety of matter suspended in it that causes the loss of visibility.

When the water is truly dirty, several things may be occurring. Surface winds stir the bottom and create suspended dirt or sand. Runoff from rain carries loose particles into the water. During runoff, it is best to avoid coves and bays and to dive upcurrent from streams and rivers or to dive elsewhere. Turbid water can also be caused by offshore currents and waves disturbing the bottom near shore. You

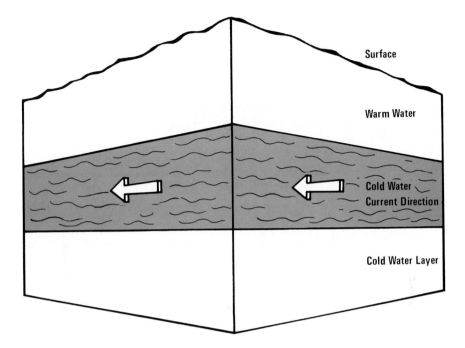

Fig. 7-2 *Thermoclines.*

find the best visibility around islands or reefs some distance from shore when visibility near the shore is low. The clearest water for diving is also located on leeward shores, away from harbors, on rocky shores with little surf, and on shores where the bottom drops quickly (Fig. 7-1).

Tidal changes in the ocean can affect visibility. When tides change drastically, the high tide disturbs much of the bottom and material far up on the beach. Extreme low tides create a layer of debris along the bottom that remains during the next high tide and limits visibility right on the bottom where you want the best visibility. Tides also move shore pollution out to sea. Before diving off coasts, you should always ask local divers about tidal conditions and check the tide tables.

Thermal (temperature) changes can also affect visibility. Cold water is denser than warm water and has a greater capacity for holding particles in suspension. Plankton, which thrives in the nutrient-rich colder waters, also tends to decrease visibility. The boundary areas between cold and warm water layers, where rapid temperature changes take place, are called *thermoclines*. In fresh water, there is usually a single thermocline. In the ocean, there may be multiple thermoclines, as well as currents within selected thermoclines. When passing through a thermocline from warmer to colder water, your ability to see may be reduced dramatically. Therefore, the consideration of water temperature changes at depth should be an important part of your dive planning (Fig. 7-2).

Any form of pollution also creates turbidity (Fig. 7-3). The pollution may stem from sewage outlets, chemical spills, drainage from a variety of outflows, or dredging in the immediate area. Rivers generally produce significant amounts of silt, either when they spill into freshwater lakes or into the ocean. Rivers also carry a great deal of suspended matter, such as microscopic life forms.

Strong surface winds can also cause currents strong enough to mix layers of water. A wind blowing in the right direction can make surface waters flow away from shore and colder bottom waters replace them. This phenomenon is called *upwelling*. Because of nutrient-rich waters rising from the bottom, upwellings are often associated with huge increases in the plankton population, and corresponding decreases in visibility.

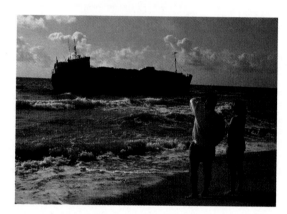

Fig. 7-3 Water may be polluted by a variety of man-made sources including effluent, runoff, ships sinking, and ships running aground as seen here. (Courtesy of Mary Brooks.)

Life Forms

Turbidity in both fresh water and salt water is not only caused by suspended dirt; it can also be caused by suspended microscopic life forms. Water containing these life forms can create the illusion of being perfectly clear from the surface; however, when you dive in it, you are unable to see because the tiny organisms reflect and scatter the light. This makes the water appear "dirty."

FRESH WATER

In fresh water, the life forms are primarily algae. Algae resemble freshwater plankton. The quantity of algae or freshwater plankton varies according to the time of the year. Generally, right after the spring thaw or before the sun warms the water in the summer, fresh water contains few if any algae. As the summer progresses, the water warms, the algae grow, and the life forms increase. This decreases visibility. As the water cools in the fall, the life forms begin to die; during the winter, they disappear.

SALT WATER

The seas are rich with plankton. The amount of plankton affecting visibility varies from day to day, season to season, and year to year. When plankton increases dramatically (a *plankton bloom*) visibility may be decreased and diving may become impossible.

Diving in Turbid Water

You need to consider three things when you dive in turbid water: visibility, direction control, and the dive plan.

Visibility

Decreased visibility affects not only how far you can see, it also affects the amount of light that penetrates the water. However, you can still see better in limited visibility water when the most sunlight is available. Because light is absorbed quite rapidly at any depth over a few feet, particularly in fresh water, you may need to use an underwater light, as shown in Fig. 7-4. However, depending on the amount of suspended matter in the water, the light may be of little value, primarily because the light hits particles of suspended matter and is reflected off at an angle equal to the approach angle (Fig. 7-5). This is sometimes called *scatter*. It affects your vision because it prevents the light from travelling very far and because there is little reflected light coming back to your eyes.

To make the underwater light useful in turbid water, you need to know how to hold it. On land, of course, you simply hold the light in the most comfortable posi-

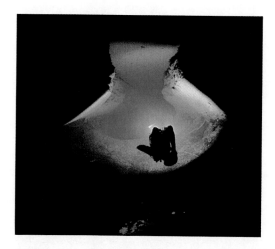

Fig. 7-4 *Use of an underwater light. (Courtesy of Jeff Bozanic.)*

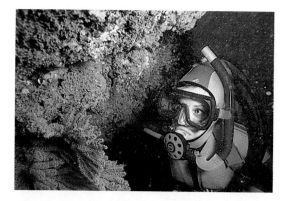

Fig. 7-5 *Scatter. (Courtesy of Jeff Bozanic.)*

tion and point it directly at an object. When you are underwater, however, you must hold the light so the reflections from the particles are scattered in directions that do not affect your ability to see. The best position, as shown in Figure 7-6, is to hold the light either above or to the side of the object. This lets the light reflect off both the suspended matter and the object itself, while giving you maximum illumination.

Fig. 7-6 Proper position for holding a light.

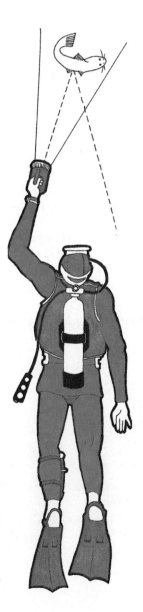

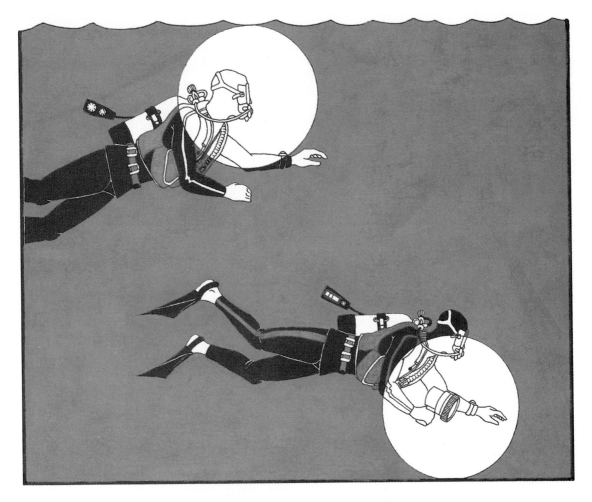

Fig. 7-7 *Vision range with underwater light.*

In turbid water, the underwater light only replaces lost surface light in the *immediate* vicinity. If visibility prevents vision beyond a few inches or feet, the light may increase your ability to perceive objects within that limit, but it does not extend your vision range beyond what the turbidity permits (Fig. 7-7).

Disorientation

The ability of the human body to function correctly and precisely depends partly upon your ability to correctly determine your position relative to the earth. This is especially important in diving. The sensations used to maintain balance are primarily from the eyes, the nerve endings in the muscles and around the joints, and certain tiny balance organs in the inner ear structure.

When you enter turbid water, you can no longer perceive the usual visual references. Subsequently, you are unable to tell "which end is up" from your nerve endings' sensations and from your balance organs' signals. This is because these nerve endings and balance organs depend, for the most part, on a correct orientation to the pull of gravity, and underwater they may not be oriented in the same direction as gravity. The brain struggles to decipher signals sent from the senses, but without the clue normally supplied by vision, incorrect or conflicting interpretations may result.

Disorientation is intensified when sunlight comes through the water and bounces off the particles, as shown in Fig. 7-8. When this occurs, the light seems to concentrate along a very narrow path, causing tunnel vision. This can distort your vision and can affect how your eyes focus, as well as affecting your peripheral vision. When you have a false sensation that you or objects around you are whirling or spinning, you may be suffering from a condition known as *vertigo*. It can increase your stress level; cause unreasonable fear, and, occasionally, result in nausea.

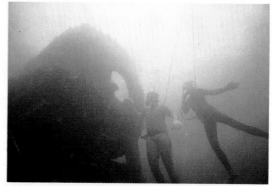

Fig. 7-8 Sun bouncing off suspended particles.

Tunnel vision and vertigo should be overcome as quickly as possible. Tunnel vision can be controlled by shutting your eyes for a moment, which relieves the disorientating effect of the light rays. You may be able to overcome vertigo by resuming an upright posture. Remember, bubbles up! Another solution to both problems is to find the bottom or any stable object to hold on to. You also can surface by using the anchor line, compass, bubbles, bottom, depth gauge, or buddy as references.

Use slight positive buoyancy when you surface, but be very careful since it is particularly difficult to judge your rate of ascent in limited visibility situations.

Direction Control
DESCENDING

Descending into dirty, dark water the first time can cause anxiety among even the most experienced divers (Fig. 7-9). Knowing the area prior to diving is an important aspect of being comfortable. Descending through turbid water can be discon-

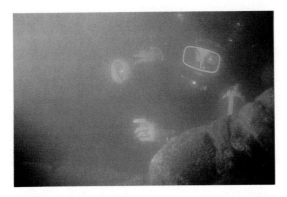

Fig. 7-9 *Limited visibility.*

certing in several ways. You must use all your senses to determine how fast you are descending and how deep you are and to generally keep the descent in perspective. It requires a keen sense of your surroundings.

Light from the surface dims quite rapidly as you begin to descend. In most cases, the temperature also changes. The change in temperature may not be very extreme, depending on the time of year and the area. The increase in pressure in your ears and around your mask also indicates descent. Even your exhalations sound different. Of course, you can always tell you are descending by watching your depth gauge. A small weighted object hung from a strap and bubbles can also indicate up and down directions.

Another way to eliminate the question of "which way is up," is by using ascent and descent lines. You do not necessarily need them when diving from shore in shallow water. However, they are recommended for low visibility diving from boats or other fixed objects (platforms) in deeper water.

You can control the rate of descent by being aware of how quickly your senses change, and by controlling buoyancy. Start by having neutral buoyancy (no air in your buoyancy compensator [BC]). To descend slowly, you should use the descent line as a guide and follow the line until you reach bottom. By remaining calm and relaxed and not descending into depths that cause discomfort, you can descend with few, if any, problems.

Horizontal Direction Control

The best and quite often the *only* way to maintain horizontal direction control on the bottom is with a compass. This is particularly true in fresh water where the bottom may be mud or plain sand with no distinguishing characteristics. You need to be skilled in compass use and have confidence in your ability to navigate with this instrument when you dive in turbid water. Your senses occasionally indicate that you should proceed in a direction when the compass says otherwise. It takes real discipline to believe in and depend on the compass.

It is important to remember, though, that your compass may be relatively useless when diving around wrecks or other metal debris. Even in fresh water diving, be careful when and where you take your compass readings as some interesting dive sites in reservoirs include old railroad trackage that might distort your compass readings.

Natural Direction Finders

In addition to the compass and dive plan, you must have a well-tuned sense of natural direction, and knowledge of natural direction finders. There are several methods to help you locate position without a compass.

1. Follow a ledge for a predetermined time, then turn around and follow it back.
2. Remember bottom features, such as rocks, coral, ravines, or ledges.
3. Move along a slope to the left, and return with the slope on the right.
4. Be aware of the shape of the bottom and know that ripples on the bottom generally run parallel to the shore (Fig. 7-10).
5. Determine the relative direction of the sun or the moon if the extent of turbidity allows it.
6. Remember the direction of the current.
7. Use large plant growth, such as kelp, to observe current and depth.
8. Be aware of sudden depth changes.

Again, a general sense of the surroundings is a must. Make a mental note of everything that you see so you can remember it in the future. In fresh water, it is very important to stay off the bottom, as shown in Fig. 7-11, to avoid disturbing the silt in case you return the same way. If you do find yourself grabbing onto objects on

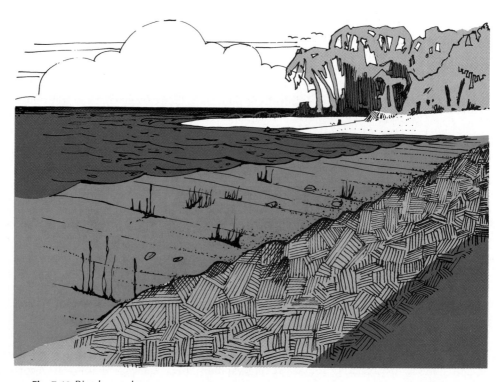

Fig. 7-10 *Ripples on bottom.*

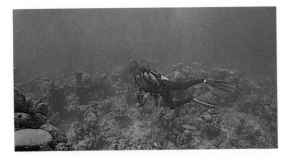

Fig. 7-11 Swimming above bottom.

the bottom, wear heavy gloves so you will not be cut on sharp objects, such as broken glass or sharp metal. Also, you should position one hand in front of you and one under your chest as you swim. This technique allows you to feel hazards with your hand first rather than making initial contact, and risking injury, with your head. Always carry a dive knife, as entanglement on fishing lines or other lines and ropes can be a problem.

ASCENDING

Before proceeding to the surface, you should establish neutral buoyancy on the bottom and confirm contact with your buddy. It is nearly impossible to tell if you are rising except by subtle physical changes in the body and the surrounding water. Consequently, you must be keenly aware of the physical changes. Pay attention to any increase in light and warmth in the water. As you ascend, the buoyancy control device will begin to inflate and your ascent rate will increase.

Release the air in the BC to reduce the ascent rate to an acceptable level. Once you begin to ascend in turbid water, you should continue all the way to the surface. Remember to keep one hand overhead and to control the deflator valve to avoid hitting obstructions above you and control an out-of-control ascent.

Dive Planning

There are several components to good dive planning. One of the major ones is buddy responsibility. This begins with thoroughly knowing your buddy's gear as well as your own, including the location of buckles and the position of the alternate air source; the tank size; and your buddy's general diving ability, including how well he or she can handle stress.

Because you must pay attention to so many things while diving in turbid water, stress becomes more of a possibility. You need to develop conditioned responses so you can deal with potentially stressful situations. There is little room for error. This means you need to know *before* diving exactly what you are going to do. Prior to any dive, but especially in turbid water, carefully plan your dive, as shown in Fig. 7-12. Plan your diving time based on your air consumption rate at the intended depths so you return with one-third of the air in your tank. Enter all pertinent data in your logbook before entering the water, and get into the habit of following the

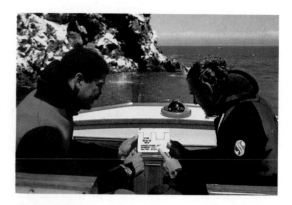

Fig. 7-12 *Dive planning.*

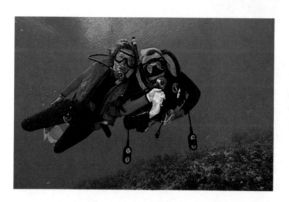

Fig. 7-13 *Technique for staying together by holding hands. (Courtesy of Mary Brooks.)*

dive plan as closely as possible. Avoiding problems under stress involves proper training, repetition of good habits, and early recognition of potential problems.

BUDDY TECHNIQUES

When you dive in limited visibility conditions, it is necessary to frequently check with your buddy. You should always be able to see your buddy or be within reach. If you find it hard to stay together, hold hands, hold your buddy's tank harness, or use a buddy line (Fig. 7-13). However, you and your buddy must agree before the dive on what procedure to use if you become separated. In this situation, you should immediately attempt to locate your buddy. Stop and listen for breathing sounds or other signals your buddy might attempt to make. If location has not been made after 1 minute, rejoin on the surface. If you still have not found each other, initiate your emergency plan.

ACTIVITIES IN TURBID WATER

Virtually every activity that can be done in clear water can be done in limited visibility. Photography, for example, involves taking closeups instead of panoramic shots (Fig. 7-14). Explorers can concentrate on small areas. Collecting artifacts is another good activity for turbid water. The closer range of vision lets you see objects you might otherwise miss.

Water at Night

The underwater world at night is truly special. After sunset, both fresh and salt water are usually calmer and more serene than during the day. Yet, this environment is exciting because the darkness gives you a narrowed field of vision; it takes longer than normal to inspect each nook and cranny. You can experience new sensations and life forms. Your artificial light illuminates brilliant colors, and objects appear even nearer and larger than they do during the day.

Life Forms

Many different species of animals are active at night. This is the best time for them to feed without being threatened by their natural enemies. Since the darkness provides them with a protective cloak, these nocturnal creatures tend to be tame. Some allow you to touch them; whereas during the day, you are fortunate to even see them (Fig. 7-15). Many of these creatures are drawn to your underwater light like magnets. The hypnotic effect of the light also makes them easy to touch.

One unique characteristic of the water at night is bioluminescence, the emission of light from millions of tiny planktonic organisms that inhabit the water. When this phenomenon occurs, any movement in the water creates a blue-green glow. Creatures, including humans, swim along and you can witness their phosphorescent trails. When you turn off your light, your own body even glows in the dark as you move.

Fig. 7-14 Close-up photography.

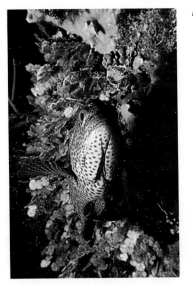

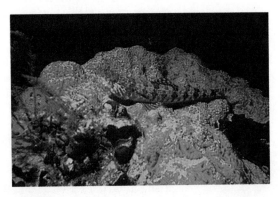

Fig. 7-15 Tame night creatures.

Night Diving

While night diving is undoubtedly quite spectacular, it also contains an element of danger. To minimize that danger, it is essential to not dive in an area that is completely unfamiliar to you. Dive in an area either you or your buddy has seen in the daytime, and preferably an area with which you are both familiar. Ideally, the area you choose for night diving should have easy access, be rather shallow, and have a good reef formation. Heavy surf, offshore reefs, and thick kelp should be avoided at night. If you cannot dive from a boat, choose a night diving spot that protects you from the surf, tidal changes, and other strong water movement. Bays and peninsulas are usually good for diving from the shore.

You also should be aware of other conditions. The water should be clear. Know the visibility probability. It is very unwise to dive in low visibility at night. Know what the bottom is like; whether it is rocky, sand, or muddy. Determine the maximum depth you intend to go and do not exceed that limit.

Tow a float and maintain contact with your buddy. Chemical light sticks make it easier to maintain contact or locate temporarily lost divers.

You should be aware of the marine life you will probably see. While it is unlikely any harmful creatures will be in the vicinity, it is not impossible. Being aware of how they may react to divers and underwater lights can prepare you and help you avoid any possible confrontation. Make sure the dive is enjoyable by removing all undue stress and unnecessary hazards before you dive.

Night diving is safe when you take all the necessary precautions to eliminate errors. It is an activity for people who are capable in the water and confident of their ability. It is *not* an activity for people who are claustrophobic, who fear the dark, or who are at all unsure of their diving skills.

Equipment

Night diving requires that you have more thorough equipment knowledge than is needed in daytime limited visibility diving. You need enough good equipment to dive safely, in addition to proper gear preparation.

Equipment required for any dive, especially at night, begins with the BC. Neutral buoyancy control is absolutely essential at night, particularly in fresh water, so you can stay off the bottom and avoid stirring it more than necessary. You should have a power inflator on your BC to ensure positive control without needing to use both hands to inflate it orally. An alternate air source is a must.

You need to carry a whistle. If you and your buddy become separated on the surface or underwater, or if you lose your light source, the whistle can be used to reunite you. Search teams may also use whistles to locate lost divers. The diving knife is necessary for diving at night. It should be within your immediate reach, as well as being sharp, so you can quickly free yourself of any lines or rope. Gloves are as much a requirement for night diving as they are for diving in turbid water. They protect you from cutting yourself on sharp objects that cannot be seen at night.

The compass is an essential piece of safety equipment for night diving as well as diving in turbid water during the day. It points the way back to the entry point, be it on the boat or on the shore.

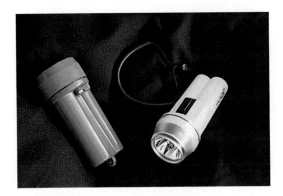

Fig. 7-16 Small night-diving lights.

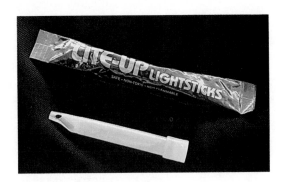

Fig. 7-17 Chemical glow lights.

Equipment Preparation

Go over all your gear and make sure everything is correctly adjusted before leaving for the dive site. It is difficult to dress and adjust your equipment in the dark. Poorly adjusted gear also creates unnecessary stress that can result in problems. Specifically, adjust your fins so they fit over the wet suit boots and secure the straps. Make sure your weight belt has exactly the correct amount of weight and that the weights are properly located and secured. Check all straps on every piece of equipment and make sure they are the correct length and are set exactly to the correct size. In short, be sure everything about your equipment is right and know where everything is located.

Underwater Lights

The most essential additional piece of equipment for night diving is obviously the underwater light. Before selecting a light you must first know how you intend to use it. Lights range from small night diving lights (Fig. 7-16), small chemical glow lights (Fig. 7-17), to large lights (Fig. 7-18). The uses for these lights vary; it is not inconceivable that you may want a combination of lights for any given dive to assure safety. Small powerful strobes are useful for additional illumination.

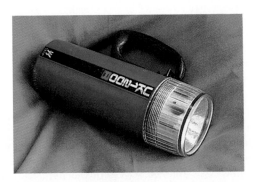

Fig. 7-18 Large underwater light.

The small lights are generally used as backup or safety lights or to carry during the daytime for casual observation under rocks and into tight places. Another safety light is the chemical light. It is preferred to the strobe light because it provides a constant visible light, which will glow for several hours. You should carry it on your body so your location is obvious to your buddy. Many divers attach the chemical light to the tank valve using a tie wrap.

Rechargeable lights are powered by a nickel-cadmium battery pack, which may be recharged by plugging it into a wall socket. They have up to 100,000 or more candlepower and are certainly the best general light for night diving.

There are even larger lights available that use lead-acid or similar batteries and illuminate a greater area than the lights previously mentioned. These lights, however, are primarily used for very clear water. They also are expensive and are somewhat awkward to use, except for very capable divers.

When you find the light suitable for your needs, it is essential to check several other features.

1. Check the light output and beam angle in a darkened room. You need narrower beams for more penetration of light and wider beams for close-up work.
2. The case surrounding the light itself should be durable.
3. The "O" ring seal must be positive and stable.
4. You should be able to hold and operate the light in one hand while you are wearing gloves.
5. The switch should have a lock to prevent the light from accidentally turning on when not in use.
6. Check to see how long the light takes to completely recharge.
7. The light should have a manufacturer's guarantee.

LIGHT PREPARATION

In preparing your light for a night dive, first make sure the batteries are completely charged, if they are of the rechargeable type, or that the light has new batteries. Next, you should clean and lubricate the light. This begins with cleaning the "O" rings and making sure they are free of defects and have been properly relubricated (Fig. 7-19). Next clean the "O" ring lands and see if there is a proper seat. Then clean and check the contacts on the light, as shown in Fig. 7-20, and check for good electrical continuity. Reseal the light to make sure it is leakproof.

Once you have reassembled the light and are sure it is working properly, check the lanyard. The light is attached to the wrist by the lanyard so you cannot lose the light if you drop it. It should be adjustable and secure (Fig. 7-21).

USING THE UNDERWATER LIGHT

The underwater light is simple to use. Unlike limited visibility diving in the daytime, you can point the light directly at the object you want to illuminate. You and your buddy should designate a system of signalling with lights. For example, to gain your buddy's attention, you may want to flash the light back and forth or turn

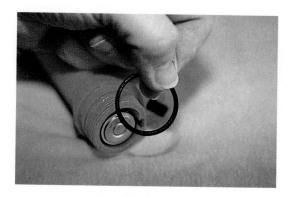

Fig. 7-19 *"O" ring inspection and lubrication.*

Fig. 7-20 *Inspection of contacts on light.*

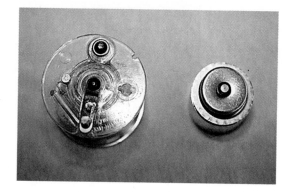

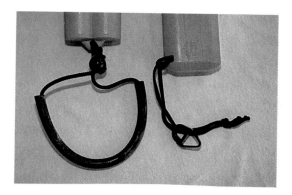

Fig. 7-21 *Lanyard attached to a light.*

the light on and off. However, you should never shine the light in your buddy's eyes.

For safety purposes, you and your buddy should each have two lights and under no circumstances should either one of you dive without a light. With both of you having a second light as a backup, you are left with three lights should one burn out. This should give you a large enough safety margin to continue the dive.

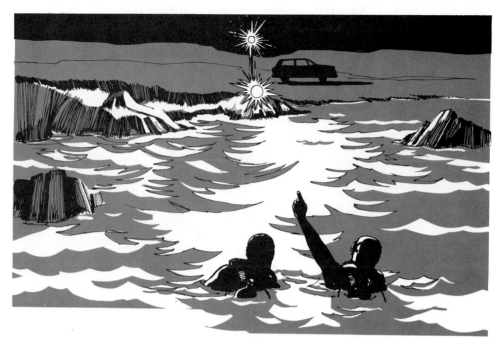

Fig. 7-22 *Light at entry point.*

If in an extreme case all lights are lost, hold hands with your buddy and establish positive buoyancy before leaving the bottom. Monitor your ascent rate and carefully ascend to the surface.

Directional Control
ENTERING

When diving from shore, it is essential to have a light at your entry point, as shown in Fig. 7-22. This light not only helps you on entry, it also is a landmark to swim toward on your return. You may want to use permanent lights that you know will still be on when you end the dive, such as street lights. You may want to align these with auxiliary lights to show which direction to exit. Auxiliary lights include flashers, strobe lights, certain types of lanterns, or roadside barricade flashers. Make sure any flashing lights you use are permitted on the beach.

The best type of auxiliary light to use is one that lights a wide area. This makes both the entry and the exit considerably safer and gives a constant shore beacon you can see if you need to surface for orientation. When you use auxiliary lights, it is wise to have someone there to guard your light, especially if it is your only means of orienting yourself after the dive.

Prior to entering the water, again check your buddy's gear as well as your own. Agree once again on your dive plan, and take a compass reading in the direction you want to go. Then enter together and descend together or at least until you can see each other. Do not begin the actual dive until you have joined and are prepared to move on the bottom.

When diving from a boat at night, use the normal entry, but try to enter as quietly as possible to avoid disturbing the aquatic life. This type of entry is also much safer than plunging into dark water where there may be hidden obstacles.

UNDERWATER DIRECTION CONTROL

You and your buddy should move along the bottom to the dive site, as opposed to moving on the surface. This naturally depends on conditions and the nature of the dive. A general rule, however, is to keep the dive within a reasonably limited distance from your entry point. By following this rule, you will find that moving along the bottom to the actual dive site is preferable.

As previously mentioned, there is an interesting phenomenon that takes place at night when you are away from shore or underwater. The limits of visibility do not allow you to see a wide enough area for geographic orientation, so it becomes nearly impossible to tell direction without moving directly along a coral head, ledge, or the bottom slope. On a flat, muddy bottom, it becomes virtually impossible to tell where you are and in what direction you are going. For these reasons, you should use the compass.

Direction control is much easier if you have a surface float with a light, ascent/descent line, diving flag, and anchor. You use the light as a reference for ascending and descending.

EXITING

With the light at the entry point illuminating enough of the area, you can expect a safe exit. Use the normal procedure for exiting, but be particularly alert for hidden hazards below the surface at the exit point. Pick a safe exit point where you can avoid areas of sharp coral, beds of sea urchins, sharp rocks, or other hazards.

Dive Planning

A great deal has been said about the value of a dive plan. It is a point that can hardly be stressed enough, particularly for night diving. It is important that you follow an exact procedure because the continuity of the plan establishes the highest probability of safety.

BUDDY TECHNIQUES

The buddy techniques for diving in turbid water and at night are generally the same. While diving, you need to monitor your buddy's attitude. Be certain your buddy is comfortable, is moving smoothly and in a relaxed way, and is under control. Remember, the greatest potential for trouble is accidental separation. Buddy diving is dependent upon a mutual agreement to follow certain procedures and a dive plan. Both members of the buddy pair must be willing and able to make this commitment, and this willingness reaches its peak when diving in limited visibility conditions or at night.

Should separation occur, the procedure is much the same as for any limited visibility situation. Both you and your buddy should make two quick revolutions and attempt to rejoin. Look for your buddy's light and, at the same time, shine your light directly outward so it might cast its glare on your diving partner. If there is not contact after 30 seconds, go directly to the surface and rejoin. Should your buddy fail to come to the surface within 30 seconds, wait no more than another 30 seconds while looking for bubbles, and then immediately initiate a search.

NIGHT DIVING ACTIVITIES

Most any underwater activity that can be enjoyed during the day can also be pleasant at night. But there are some particularly outstanding activities. One of those is photography. During the daytime when lights are unnecessary, the eye perceives color depending on the depth of the dive. At night, however, the sun is replaced by the artificial light, which brings out those special and spectacular colors that simply do not show up during the day. Of course, there is the new dimension of the additional creatures that appear at night. Night provides an excellent opportunity for you to study shy and interesting creatures and for exploration.

As you continue limited visibility diving, you may find that when you dive in clear water, your navigation skills, buoyancy control methods, and buddy system techniques have improved. You may also discover an increased sensitivity to your surroundings. By following these guidelines for diving in turbid water and at night, you can be in control of each dive, which enables you to routinely deal with problems and continue with your main objective—to enjoy the dive.

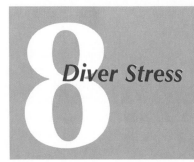

8 *Diver Stress*

KEY TERMS

Stress	Pre-dive stress	Task loading
Pregnancy	Patent foramen ovale	Fatigue
Out-of-air situations	Over-weighting	Orientation
Limitations	Panic	

The psychology of diving deals mainly with diver stress. Stress is defined as "a physical, chemical, or emotional factor that causes bodily or mental tension." Stress can be any stimulus that *disturbs* or interferes with the normal psychological state. In many ways stress makes our lives interesting and exciting. Some people thrive on such stimulation. Controlled stress adds to diving's challenge and excitement. Uncontrolled stress can lead to anxiety, panic, and injury. Most of the stress covered here is stress that detracts from diving safety. You will learn to recognize stress, to control it, and to deal with uncontrolled stress in others.

Scuba diving is a blend of both the physical and mental aspects of life as well as having definite social aspects. Diving is an enjoyable, interesting adventure. There is a great psychological value to diving that is often overlooked; that is, to get away from the negative stresses or pressures of everyday life. Diving is beneficial because it is a demanding and rewarding activity. Other psychological attributes of diving include:

1. Feeling of weightlessness underwater
2. Personal ego satisfaction or inner feelings of self-identity
3. Challenge of underwater activities
4. Freedom of the underwater world
5. Thrill of exploration, discovering new places, or seeing what few people, if any, have ever seen before
6. Excitement caused by an element of perceived risk

The reasons people dive also include the social aspects of interacting with others who share a common interest in diving and gaining satisfaction from helping or teaching others. The very special interpersonal relationship of the buddy pair is not often shared in other human activities. After diving for some time, you can gain a feeling of openness with yourself, your buddy, and the environment. After the dive, there is a feeling of well-being that is hard to describe to nondivers.

Sport diving is a demanding, yet rewarding adventure, and for many people it may be their ultimate adventure. Diving can be the very essence of those activities that add joy to your life. Yet, with all this, diving can also subject you to a variety of stressors. To diminish the risks of diving you need to understand the chain of events leading to stress, what the outcome of stress may be, and methods to gain control of stress. The central idea is to not allow stress to develop, but if it does develop in either you or another diver during a dive, you should understand how to recognize and control it.

Causes and Effects of Diver Stress

There are several physical and mental causes of diver stress. It is difficult to isolate each cause as the only factor leading to stress, for several of these usually combine to create significant stress.

Individual psychological make-up and life experience need to be considered when studying the causes and effects of diver stress. What puts one diver into a serious state of stress may leave another diver totally unconcerned and in full control of the situation.

Discussing the causes and effects of stress is not meant to discourage you from diving, but stressors are realistic and they may affect your diving. To be a competent advanced recreational diver you should become very familiar with the causes of stress so you will be able to avoid them or deal with them early in the evolution of the stress state.

PHYSICAL CAUSES

Major physical causes of diver stress include: predive stress, poor physical conditioning, task loading, and adverse environmental conditions. Any or all of these may lead to excess fatigue, equipment difficulties, over-consumption of a limited air supply, and buoyancy-related problems. Each of these needs to be viewed in relation to the others and to the impact it may have on stress when the effects of stress are studied.

Predive Stress

The time before any dive is just as important as the dive itself. The predive begins when you decide to make a dive, be it 1 day or 2 months in advance.

The time element is a big factor in producing predive stress. If your diving companions are already suited up and ready to jump in the water while you are struggling with the wet suit zipper or searching for your depth gauge, stress could obviously develop. A stressful state can, in turn, cause you to overlook crucial things, such as checking your regulator, or you may overlook a necessary piece of equipment in your rush to plunge into the water. Good dive planning and preparedness should allow enough time for a calm orderly beginning to your dive.

Poor Physical Conditioning

Diving requires good physical conditioning. If you are not in good shape, even the simplest movements or skills may cause you to go beyond your physical capabilities, and may bring on stress. Poor physical condition is not just a matter of a lack of strength but also includes any significant medical condition that affects respiration, circulation, consciousness, ability to equalize pressure, or judgment. Some conditions, which might initially disqualify someone from diving, can develop after one is certified and should then limit one's diving either temporarily or permanently. These include:

1. Heart trouble
2. Respiratory impairment
3. Epilepsy
4. Regular medication to control a serious condition
5. Ear and sinus trouble
6. Recent serious operation
7. Injury or illness

Some individuals may be excluded altogether from diving because of limiting physical conditions. Some conditions deserve special consideration when related to diving.

First, know your limitations and dive within them. A physical handicap itself does not necessarily prohibit diving, provided the diver with the handicap can dive effectively and still relate to and effect a rescue of a fellow diver. There are diving opportunities available to handicapped individuals for whom special accommodations are needed to lessen their risk of injury during diving.

Certain temporary conditions or activities, such as colds, flu, excessive drinking, use of drugs, and fatigue can render an individual temporarily unfit to dive. During the course of one's life, conditions may develop that permanently preclude further diving.

Age plays a role in diving; as you get older you may need to be more conservative in your range of diving activities. But of even more importance is your level of fitness at any age. Divers need to reevaluate themselves before each dive to decide whether or not they are fit for that particular dive.

Smoking deserves special consideration, as it significantly detracts from the fitness of the diver's respiratory system. If at all possible, divers should not smoke. Due to the fact that carbon monoxide from cigarette smoke has a greater affinity for the oxygen-carrying chemical in the blood than does oxygen, it is suggested that smokers refrain from smoking for at least 12 hours before the dive. Smokers who have recovered from a cold within the 2 weeks before a dive have a greater risk of embolism owing to the increased mucus production found in smokers and the possibility that it may increase the risk of air trapping when ascending.

Recent research indicates that women who are pregnant should not scuba dive. The key issue is not the exercise of diving, but the physiologic changes that occur under pressure, particularly as related to decompression sickness. This affects both the mother and the fetus. During pregnancy the fetus has a patent foramen ovale as a normal feature of its circulatory system, which allows any nitrogen bubbles to pass directly from the right side of the heart into the systemic circulatory system— brain, heart, and other organs. This presents a potentially dangerous condition. If they must, women should do only limited shallow diving during pregnancy, and it is best that they not dive at all.

Fatigue

Fatigue is a normal physiologic response to exercise. The positive aspects are that increased work on a consistent basis results in increased cardiovascular capacity, which can lead to increased diving performance. Negatively, fatigue and poor physical fitness are interrelated and stress can be increased secondary to fatigue. Staying in the water too long, using equipment improperly, and lacking the proper equipment, can cause you to tire quickly. Fatigue can also be caused by excess task loading. Fatigue may limit your ability to think clearly before you recognize any other signs of fatigue. This inability to think clearly may add greatly to stress.

Task Loading

A planned increase in task loading can improve performance over a period of time. When unplanned, increased task loading creates increased stress. Causes of such unplanned increased task loading may include the amount of time spent underwater or an excessive amount of work required within a given time period. The work may encompass swimming, breathing, snorkeling, making a rescue, compensating for improper weighting or buoyancy control, or any other strenuous activity. All of these add to the stress level.

Often it is the pace at which an activity is attempted that leads to the task overloading. Because hurried movements and even breathing itself require more work underwater than on land, a vicious cycle can develop if activities are paced too fast. When diving in a group or with just your buddy, the pace needs to be adjusted to the progress of the slowest diver—never expect a diver to catch up to you, as it simply creates an unnecessary task load and increased stress.

Environment

Dangerous or suddenly changing environmental conditions obviously can be major physical factors contributing to diver stress. Stress may be increased by surf conditions that are overwhelming or swimming into unnoticed powerful currents. Diving in cold water can cause additional stress. Diving at greater depths increases the work of breathing because of the increased density of gases, which adds to stress.

Stress levels may increase as the range of visibility decreases due to dirty or turbid water, night diving, or deep diving. Poor visibility also makes proper underwater orientation difficult, which causes diver discomfort and increases stress.

Certain situations that are confining or restricting to bodily movement can cause stress. In such situations, the stress results from a limited ability to move freely or the perception of being confined. Examples of these may be entanglement in kelp, weeds, lines, or nets (Fig. 8-1). Diving in caves, wrecks, or under ice adds significantly to stress and for this and other reasons requires special training. Diving equipment, necessitated by some environments, such as a dry suit or a heavy wet suit, can cause restrictions and require enhanced skills so you will be able to effectively cope with the increased level of stress.

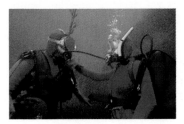

Fig. 8-1 *Entanglement is a stressful situation where the diver must control the natural response to panic.*

Threats emanating from the environment may include animals that bite, such as moray eels, barracuda, and sharks (Fig. 8-2). Each of these is a possible threat, but most often the danger from them is grossly exaggerated.

Boat propellers, boats immediately overhead on ascent, and spearguns are direct physical threats. A diver who is aware of the presence of any of these can have an increased stress load.

Any of these environmental stressors are difficult to eliminate, but with forethought and appropriate training the well-trained diver knows of their existence,

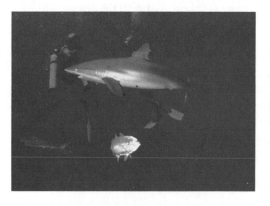
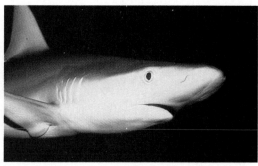

Fig. 8-2 Though not usually a threat, the presence of sharks and their reputations can be a significant stressor on divers.

understands the relative risk, and manages the potential stress through knowledge and experience.

Equipment Difficulties

Early in your diving instruction you learned that "fit and comfort" were the keys to appropriate equipment for diving. If you are not completely familiar or comfortable with the diving equipment you use on a dive, stress could possibly result. A rental buoyancy compensator (BC) could have an inflator you are not used to or may not fit properly. Your weight may not have been properly adjusted for the exposure suit you are wearing. Improperly maintained equipment may lead to a leaking BC or malfunctioning regulator, both situations that may place a diver at risk and cause unnecessary and avoidable stress.

Another potential stress factor is the lack of needed equipment. If you are forced onto a long surface swim and do not have a snorkel or you are inadequately protected for a cold dive and begin to experience hypothermia, you are exposed to physical stressors that could be eliminated with proper planning.

Air Supply and Ascents

"Running out-of-air" is associated with uncontrolled ascents leading to lung-over-pressure injuries and near-drowning. In most cases, a diver is actually just low-on-air, so these cannot really be considered "out-of-air" situations. The instinctive response to "running out-of-air" is to hold one's breath and head for the surface. "Out-of-air" emergencies produce substantial stress and put the diver at risk from air embolism and/or decompression sickness. The prevention of stress in these situations will be discussed later.

Buoyancy Control Problems

Buoyancy control problems can contribute subtly to stress. Inflated BCs produce a greater surface area to the water resulting in increased drag, which adds to the work of swimming. Over-weighting needs to be offset by BC inflation or swimming harder for the diver to achieve neutral buoyancy. With the BC inflated just moving in the water requires overcoming resistance, adding to work load and stress.

Major problems of stress associated with buoyancy happen when a diver does not have or use a buoyancy control device, when the buoyancy control device is not functioning, or a diver is markedly over-weighted. Records of fatal diving accidents show that few people inflated their own BCs or ditched their weights. The need for buoyancy compensation while submerged should be minimal since the diver should be weighted for neutral buoyancy for each diving situation.

MENTAL CAUSES

Major mental causes of diver stress include ego threat, buddy system failure, and lack of training that may lead to human error and mishaps. These causes are tied into the physical causes of stress, as well as being interrelated.

Ego Threat

Your ego may be threatened when you must retreat from a situation that is beyond your capabilities. If you are performing a certain underwater activity because of peer pressure or to prove to yourself it can be done, giving up can certainly affect your pride and bring on stress. It takes a greater degree of maturity and self-esteem to admit you cannot do a difficult task than to risk a diving accident trying to do it.

The anticipation of ridicule because of possible failure can add to stress and may occur in many different situations, including failure to enjoy the dive, make a rescue, gain personal control, or stay oriented underwater. Because other added stress from anticipated ridicule can make self-prophesied failure come true, you must learn to approach challenge with a positive attitude.

Buddy System Failure

When a diver loses contact with a buddy underwater, as shown in Fig. 8-3, or when he or she dives alone, the chances of a stressful situation developing increase. One

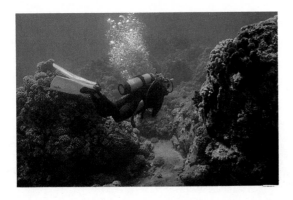

Fig. 8-3 *Loss of a buddy is an extreme stress-inducing situation.*

does not have the security of knowing someone is there to help if a problem occurs. While diving alone does not directly harm you, being alone when something goes wrong makes it difficult or sometimes impossible to deal with the situation. Part of the enhanced pleasure of diving with a buddy comes from the diminution of stress.

Lack of Training

Stress originating in training deficits can be divided into four identifiable profiles:

- Divers are certified yet poorly trained.
- Dives are made under specialty circumstances (cave, ice, wreck, or deep diving) without specialty training.
- Diving is done with new or advanced equipment without specialized instruction.
- A diver has not dived for many years and then dives without any "refresher" training.

Scuba diving can be complex and demanding, yet people still try it without proper training or supervision. The chances for stress and accidents are higher in poorly trained and uncertified divers than in those who are trained in the basic fundamentals of diving. Proper diver education also teaches how to limit exposure to negatively stressful situations and how to recognize and deal with stress, should it occur. Specialty training prepares the already certified diver for exposure to environments that otherwise might be perceived as threatening. Finally, if it has been some time since your last dive, you can get some refresher updating from a professional dive store for about the same price that it costs for the typical boat dive.

Human Error and Mishaps

Mishaps are usually the end result of a series of compounding errors or unexpected events. Each progression in the series has its own stress component and adds the stress to the next judgment or event. Poor judgment includes mistakes made before or during the dive, which have already been mentioned as sources of stress. These errors can start or add to a chain of events that becomes a mishap. Even good equipment can malfunction, environmental conditions can change unexpectedly, or other divers can force you into a stressful situation. With these unknowns, advanced training exposes you, under guidance, to situations in which your judgment can be developed. With continued diving and experience your perception and judgment will grow and your control of stress will be enhanced.

Overall Effects of Stress

The overall physical effects of stress that can be observed in a diver include:

1. Muscle tension (white knuckles)
2. Wide-eyed look (Fig. 8-4)
3. Rapid breathing
4. Rapid, jerking movements
5. Fixation or repetitive behavior

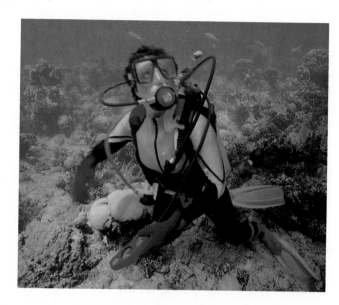

Fig. 8-4 *This is the type of look seen on the face of a diver in stress.*

In addition, many changes are happening inside the person as a reaction to stress. These cannot be observed easily by divers in the water. They include:

1. Chemical changes
2. Heart rate changes
3. Blood pressure changes
4. Increased perspiration
5. Decreased digestion

Mental changes caused by stress that another diver can observe in the water include irritability, unexpected or unusual behavior, inappropriate responses, fixation, inability to recall or use the correct action, loss of new skills, and a lack of appropriate communication with others.

All these effects of diver stress lead to additional, or cumulative, human errors, particularly in judgment. If prolonged enough, or if the diver does not gain control, stress can lead to accidents. Stress is not always a precedent for accidents, as something can happen quite unexpectedly and quickly underwater. Surprise itself can therefore create a sudden and high stress factor. The chain of events leading up to diving accidents is shown in Fig. 8-5.

Avoiding Stress

Anticipation of stress will help you avoid it. Mentally performing a task beforehand usually reduces tension and stress when the task has to be done. Any technique of avoiding stress may deal with many forms of stress. For example, gathering all the information possible about your dive and thoroughly planning it may eliminate the stresses of buddy separation, disorientation, dive termination, or emergency as-

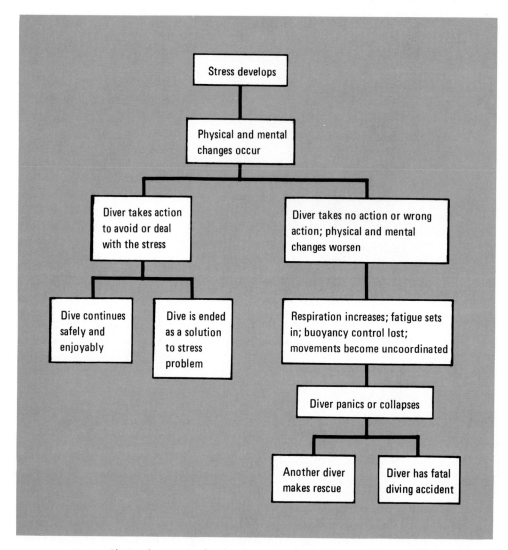

Fig. 8-5 *Chain of events in the development of stress.*

cents, to name a few. The verbalization of how you perceive an upcoming dive may change apprehension into pleasant anticipation as you share the perception of others or, as others acknowledge the legitimacy of your concerns, the dive plan may be altered or canceled. The objective is to eliminate surprise. You can gain some control over stress by being physically fit, using proper and complete equipment, being trained and experienced, and planning each dive.

PHYSICAL FITNESS

There are several ways to improve and maintain physical fitness. First, a regular medical examination is important for health care in general, not just for diving. Medical examinations should be more frequent as you become older, and the examinations should emphasize the special requirements of diving. Many diving organizations and textbooks have diving medical exam forms available.

To be physically fit, you should have adequate rest, eat a well-balanced diet, and exercise regularly. These are all particularly important for divers. The amount of rest varies significantly with each person and the amount of activity performed. Maintaining a well-balanced diet of nutritious food and avoiding foods with low or no nutritional value is a problem for many people. It is not so much a problem of understanding what is best, as it is a problem of self-discipline.

Diving is not an activity that in and of itself enhances physical conditioning to any extent, but fitness is an important preparatory part of many recreational activities. So you can be more fit for diving, your exercise should parallel the demands of diving as much as possible. Activities similar to diving that increase circulation and respiration are good, such as skin diving, snorkeling in a pool, swimming, bicycling, walking, jogging, running, and other activities that increase heart rate and breathing while utilizing leg movement.

Relaxation and recreation are important for good fitness. To be fit, you need to relieve the stress of everyday life. Other activities that contribute to relaxation and recreation also relieve stress and help you become a better diver.

Fitness immediately prior to diving is very important. There are some helpful hints that make diving more enjoyable by improving this aspect of being fit to dive as it relates to the immediate diving situation. First, you should mentally want to make the dive and be physically well. If you use regular medications and understand their side effects, you should experience no problem; however, you should still check with your physician.

You should have a good night's sleep before the dive. You need to eat well both the night before and the morning of the dive. These meals should include easily digestible foods. Exercising your eustachian tubes the night before and the morning of the dive may make equalization easier during the dive. You may either repeatedly "clear" your ears or chew gum. Moderate repeat "clearings" may make it easier for you to clear during the actual dive. Overdoing this though may force throat contents into the eustachian tubes causing irritation. So, this is another of the aspects or techniques utilized in diving that must be done in moderation. In the final analysis, gum chewing may prove to be potentially less injurious and still get the job done.

Good mental and physical fitness is a lifestyle decision that only divers can make for themselves. It can be easy to be fit, and the reward of being fit not only improves your diving, it also increases your enjoyment of life by relieving stress.

EQUIPMENT USE

You can do a great deal to help avoid stress by using proper and complete equipment. Your regulator should be a well-maintained, high-quality regulator equipped with a submersible pressure gauge, power inflator, and an alternate air source. A good BC with a power inflator from the regulator makes diving easier and, therefore, decreases stress.

Many causes of stress can be avoided by wearing a wet suit or dry suit. A wet suit jacket is recommended even in warm water. In colder water, wet suits should be thicker and more complete. In very cold water, you may wish to use a dry suit, provided you receive appropriate additional training in its use.

Your snorkel should be comfortable, with a large diameter bore and no features that will increase breathing resistance. A knife is a safety tool you should carry to deal with entanglements. Information equipment, such as depth gauges, watches, and compasses, should be used. New equipment, particularly new regulators, a new BC, or dive computers should be tested under controlled conditions in confined water, or under the supervision of an instructor before use in open water.

TRAINING AND EXPERIENCE

During your beginning diving course you "over-learned" many skills and concepts to make you a safer diver. Over-learning means doing some skill or activity so often that you do it automatically even when stressed. Now, as you continue your training in open water, with advanced or specialty courses, you continue that process. The more complex the diving, the more important it is to avoid stress and repeatedly execute appropriate responses under simulated difficult conditions (Fig. 8-6).

Experience is vital to maintaining diving skills and being fit and relaxed during diving. This experience should be gained under controlled conditions within your diving ability.

DIVE PLANNING

It is important to plan your dive with your buddy or other fellow divers prior to the actual dive. "Plan your dive—dive your plan" is a valuable concept, but it should be applied with common sense. The plan should not be so rigid that it takes the joy

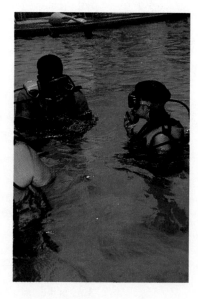

Fig. 8-6 *Additional training or refresher training is a way to become more familiar with various diving skills and more comfortable when diving.*

out of diving. The plan should be flexible enough to take advantage of opportunities or handle unanticipated situations. It should be based on the fitness and experience of the least capable diver in the team.

During the dive, you and your buddy should make reasonable modifications to ensure both safety and enjoyment. An important aspect of dive planning is that either diver can, at any time, decide not to dive, or terminate the dive based on changing medical, physical, psychological, or environmental conditions.

The dive plan should include such items as:

1. Objectives
2. Equipment
3. Environmental conditions
4. Diver fitness
5. Buddy system
6. General direction of dive
7. Exit and entry points
8. Planned depth, time, and air usage
9. How changes will be made
10. Criteria for dive termination
11. Possible stress factors
12. Hand signals
13. Emergency procedures

Dealing with Known Stresses

Much of the material just presented involves anticipating stress. You can anticipate certain changes when you enter the water (Fig. 8-7). You have little control over these changes, but you learn to adapt to them. The effects of immersion include

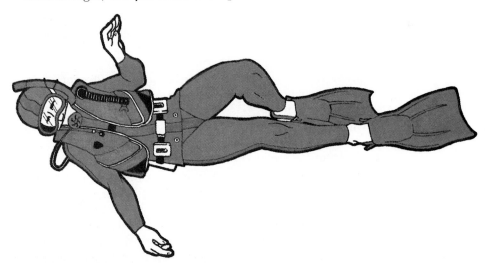

Fig. 8-7 *The diver must adapt to a multitude of changes, which add to the stress and must be understood and controlled.*

decreased heart rate, blood pressure, respiration, and temperature. However, these effects may not be felt until you have settled into the dive. Your perceived weight decreases to nearly zero. You are restricted by your wet suit, straps, and belts. The mask narrows your field of vision, while the range of visibility and color decreases. The unfamiliar surroundings and vertical dimension make it hard to orient yourself and you may feel apprehension of the unknown or unseen. Because of all these changes, at the surface and on the bottom, allow yourself time to adjust. When you feel ready to proceed, and your buddy gives the "OK" signal, start the dive in a slow, easy manner. You should always function within the environment and not attempt to overcome it.

Breathing, Moving, and Orientation

Techniques in breathing, moving, and orientation are interrelated and involve the skills of swimming, snorkeling, buoyancy control, navigation, breathing, and ascents. Each will be presented as it relates to stress reduction.

Breathing takes work and uses energy; it becomes more difficult if you go deeper or work harder and stress increases. The easiest way to breath is through your mouth at the surface. The next easiest way is through the regulator and the least easiest is through the snorkel. The snorkel is used to aid surface swimming. The design has improved greatly, but snorkeling is still the most difficult way to breath. All divers should carry and use a snorkel, but there are excellent ways to avoid using it as often, thereby decreasing the work and stress of diving.

A good way to decrease snorkel use is to use a compass for underwater navigation so you can arrive at your exit point without a long surface swim. Sometimes you can swim on your back on the surface, relaxing with your BC floating you and breathing through your mouth. A compass bearing or visual range can help keep you on course in this position and you can periodically look over your shoulder as a check. When surface conditions are rough the regulator should be used instead of the snorkel and even in calm water some of your remaining air can be used for the exit swim.

Although it is usually easy to breath from a regulator, regulator breathing can be stressful at times. Regulators are high-quality pieces of equipment, but it is possible to demand too much air from them. Regulators perform at less than maximum capacity when tank pressure is 500 psi or less, at a depth of 100 feet or more, when you have a rapid breathing rate, or when the regulator is poorly maintained (Fig. 8-8). To reduce the work and stress of diving, select a high quality regulator and have it professionally serviced every year. In addition, avoid deep diving, hold at least 500 psi in reserve, and breath in a slow, deep, relaxed manner.

Swimming with fins is work and this may increase the stress level. You should use fins as efficiently as possible, with strong, full, slow kicks from the hips with the knees "unlocked" while you point your toes. Other styles such as the dolphin kick should be used periodically to alternate and rest muscle groups. This reduces fatigue.

Swimming can be lessened if you descend and ascend with good buoyancy control, as shown in Fig. 8-9. Proper weighting and good neutral buoyancy, of course,

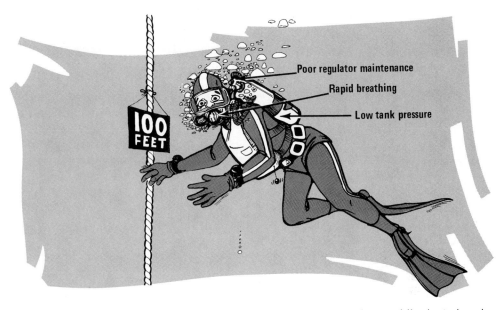

Poor regulator maintenance
Rapid breathing
Low tank pressure

Fig. 8-8 *Stress can be induced by poor regulator performance leading to difficulty in breathing at depth.*

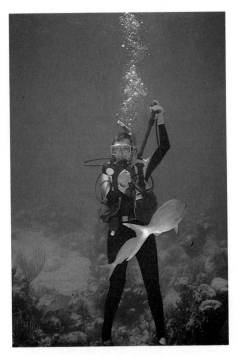

Fig. 8-9 *The diver can make mid-water buoyancy adjustments to reduce the work of swimming and stress connected with a dive.*

reduce the work of swimming during the dive. Hands and fins can be used to pull or push along the bottom. This bottom crawling technique depends on the nature of the bottom and should always be tempered with respect for the environment.

Any reduced air situations can be stressful. Approaches to getting out of the situation can be less stressful if options are understood and necessary skills practiced. If faced with a "low-on-air" or "out-of-air" situation, a normal ascent is the best option whenever possible. If air supply allows, a diver should stop, breathe easy, and then swim to the surface in a controlled manner. The next option is to ascend using your buddy's alternate air source. The alternate air source is a good ascent choice when your buddy is closer than the surface or when there is an obstruction to the surface (ice, cave, wreck, or heavy kelp).

If needs are more urgent, an option is the emergency swimming ascent performed as closely to a normal ascent as possible. This includes looking up, regulator in mouth, swimming a bit faster, and exhaling more and inhaling less to keep lungs at as near normal volume as possible. An even more demanding option is a buoyant ascent done by ditching weights and/or inflating the BC. This is done like an emergency swimming ascent, but it is faster.

As an acknowledged high risk option, and when no other method is available, a buddy breathing ascent can be used, as shown in Fig. 8-10. "Out-of-air" ascents will be rare if you use submersible pressure gauges, maintain air reserves, have alternate air sources, use the buddy system and dive planning, develop relaxed breathing, good fitness, buoyancy control, and dive within your limitations.

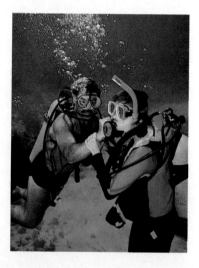

Fig. 8-10 *The buddy breathing ascent is the least attractive air sharing technique due to the stress-load connected with the complexity of the skill in an emergency situation.*

By carefully planning your dive, diving your plan, and monitoring your remaining air, your ascent will be made with plenty of reserve air and energy. Enhancing efficiency is easy. Use and carry only the necessary equipment. Keep your equipment as simple and streamlined as possible, and swim slowly while staying completely underwater. You can decrease the drag created by equipment, especially the BC, if you weight yourself properly. You should weight yourself for the shallowest depth of the dive and be able to hover at a 10- to 20-foot depth for a 3- to 5-minute precautionary stop at the end of the dive. When weighted thus, you will be able to maintain neutral or slightly negative buoyancy with as little air as possible in the BC. With minimal air in the BC your body will be more horizontal in the water and create less drag. Being properly weighted also makes the ascent itself simpler. It is much easier to control buoyancy during the ascent when you have less expanding air in the buoyancy control device (Fig. 8-11).

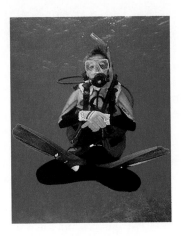

Fig. 8-11 *This diver has been properly weighted for neutral buoyancy. Proper weighting and good buoyancy control significantly reduces stress.*

Orientation is extremely important in the three-dimensional underwater world. To deal with and avoid stress, follow the bottom contour or an anchor line, swim a compass course, watch your bubbles, or your buddy, use buoyancy, and check your depth gauge. Each, or better, several of these methods can give you a sense of location and orientation in the watery inner space. This, in turn, decreases the stress level.

Buddy Diving

Buddy diving has already been mentioned as a means of reducing stress. However, buddy diving itself can contribute to stress unless certain parameters are met in buddy selection and communication. Buddy diving's goal is twofold: (1) enhance the enjoyment by sharing experiences, and (2) decrease the risk by sharing responsibilities.

As your diving progresses, you will find your criteria for selecting a buddy changes somewhat. If you are a very skilled diver who is doing deeper dives or are involved in photography, you will not be at ease with a novice diver, nor will the novice be at ease in your diving environment. In order to buddy dive more comfortably, select a partner who shares your abilities and interests.

If a diver is a totally new buddy to you, take the time to get to know the individual. Share your diving background and demonstrate how your equipment functions. A new buddy will usually reciprocate without feeling interrogated. Hands-on familiarity with a buddy's gear is best as is visual confirmation of air supply. Never

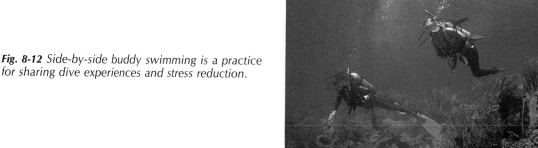

Fig. 8-12 *Side-by-side buddy swimming is a practice for sharing dive experiences and stress reduction.*

be reluctant to voice your own misgivings about any planned dive. It is much easier to change things before the dive starts.

Once in the water, dive side-by-side, staying on the same side of your buddy as much as possible, as shown in Fig. 8-12. Agree on a direction and continue in that direction until you both agree to change. Go slowly, look around, and listen for your buddy's bubbles. Share your discoveries and communicate as you go. If visibility is poor, use a buddy line or hold hands. It is reassuring to have physical contact with your buddy.

Buddy teams are commonly made of two people but, in some circumstances, other numbers are possible. In accommodating handicapped divers, threesomes are sometimes required so that two able-bodied divers can assist the handicapped diver. In other situations the handicapped diver can be one of a two-member dive team. Regardless of the arrangement, there must always be at least one able-bodied diver available when any one of the others is incapacitated. Diving in threesomes takes extra effort to stay together and should be avoided whenever possible.

If you become separated, stop, look, and listen. If you have not found your buddy, swim in a circle toward the side your buddy was on. If you still have not found your buddy, go up a few feet and turn 360 degrees looking for signs of your buddy, look up, look down, and then surface and wait for about 1 additional minute. If you both use the same procedure, your buddy should join you on the surface shortly. If this does not occur, there is cause for concern and others should be alerted about your missing buddy.

Limitations

"Know your limits and dive within them" is an excellent concept. Recreational dives should not test the limits of either you or your buddy. If you discover your limits by exceeding them in open water, you will be in an unsafe situation. When either you or your buddy is cold, tired, getting low on air, not feeling well, having difficulty, injured, uncomfortable, under undue stress, or not having a good time, you should both leave the water—diving is no longer enjoyable and is a greater risk.

When the decision has been made to end the dive, do not rush to get out of the water. Rushing will increase stress and may lead to problems during the swim back. First, stop, breath easy, and check the situation; then proceed slowly and easily. Use your equipment skillfully to make the trip as easy as possible.

Treating Symptoms

If your buddy is experiencing physical or mental symptoms of stress, you need to break the chain of events, as shown previously in Fig. 8-6. Serious accidents can often be averted by early intervention. People have a survival instinct that provides a drive to escape difficult situations. But this survival instinct may cause the wrong decision if quickly going to the surface is the automatic response.

The symptoms of stress should be treated as soon as recognized. The crucial elements in dealing with stress are: stop, breath easy, think, and get control. Additional steps are:

1. Maintain orientation
2. Control buoyancy
3. Use equipment to help
4. Use the buddy system
5. Solve the problem when under control
6. Continue slowly in the easiest possible manner.

Often the best place to solve a problem is underwater. Do not get caught in the trap of thinking that going to the surface is always necessary; often it only delays a solution and increases risk. If you are already on the surface, use positive buoyancy to help you. Maintaining control is the all-important aspect in dealing with diver stress. Loss of control leads to panic and accidents.

Loss of Control

If a diver does not recognize the causes and effects of stress so he or she can avoid or deal with it, stress may lead to the total loss of control, which is panic. Panic is a sudden unreasoning fear that causes the diver to take inappropriate action in dealing with the situation. The causes and effects of panic are extensions of stress behavior. Panic can be thought of as an acute uncontrolled behavior caused by stress, with exaggeration on the inappropriate behavior and errors in judgment.

When a distressed diver cannot regain control it may now be necessary for the diving buddy or another responsible diver to rescue the panicked diver. In this case, another person takes a risk to help someone who has allowed stress to go too far. You can significantly lessen the chance of panic by watching for early physical and mental signs of stress in yourself and in your fellow divers.

Discipline your thinking to recognize and solve problems instead of worrying about them. Develop self-control in your thinking with both training and practice. Concentrate on those parts of a problem that are important and ignore the emotional consequences. In this way, you can effectively handle stress in yourself and others. As an advanced diver, seek rescue training to enhance your skills and learn methods of dealing with panicked divers.

9 *Diver Rescue*

OBJECTIVES

At the conclusion of this chapter you should be able to:

1. Name some of the complications that may be encountered in effecting a rescue.

2. Explain how, if you are called upon to assist another diver or rescue a diver, you will be able to competently complete the rescue without becoming exhausted.

3. Describe some of the equipment concerns that should be taken into consideration during diver rescues.

4. Name the first line of defense of diving difficulties.

5. Name some of the steps relative to everyday diving that can lead to prevention or are means of self-rescue.

6. Explain the concept of buddy assist.

7. Describe skills that might be employed in the buddy assist or buddy rescue.

8. Define the meaning of and need for diving rescues.

9. Name the first step in a diving rescue once you have made contact with the distressed diver.

10. Describe the types of tows utilized to assist fatigued divers.

KEY TERMS

Margin of safety

Prevention

Buddy assist

Mouth-to-mask breathing

Do-si-do assist

Self-rescue

Cramp relief

First-aid

Mouth-to-snorkel ventilation

Shock

Sprains, strains, fractures

Pacing

Tank-cradle technique

Fin push assist

Survival swimming techniques

Buddy rescue

CPR

Tank pull assist

Oxygen system

Marine life injuries

Wounds

Splinting

Many of the reasons and methods for diver rescue come from studying the effects of stress. Understanding the causes of stress that may lead to accidents is a large part of diver rescue. Avoiding and dealing with stress are the very essence of accident prevention; this makes diver rescues unnecessary. Finally, the deterioration of a diver's situation to a point where he or she can no longer continue functioning, is the time when diver rescue becomes all-important.

The greatest value in mastering diver rescue is to you personally. The knowledge and skills of diver rescue make you a better, more confident, and capable diver who is able to help yourself and avoid trouble. The intention of this chapter is not to make you a diving lifeguard or member of a search and recovery team, but to help you be a more responsible diver and buddy. Still, someday, your rescue skills may be used to help another diver other than your buddy, or even to help a non-diver.

Rescue Considerations
ENVIRONMENT

The remarkably diverse, demanding, and interesting diving environment adds greatly to your enjoyment of diving, but during a diving rescue the environment may make the rescue more difficult.

Diving accidents often occur far from the shore or boat, in deep water, or in poor visibility. The water may be moving with surge, surf, surface chop, or currents. Caves, ice, wrecks, or kelp may restrict movement and coral or other aquatic growth may make it difficult to leave the water. The water may be cold and, therefore, drain your energy. Accidents can occur underwater or on the surface. These diverse environmental conditions can usually be handled if you are trained and if you operate within reasonable limits. Difficult environmental conditions clearly show why you need a "margin of safety," a reserve of energy for rescues made at these times. The rescue procedures and skills detailed later provide ways to deal with these conditions.

COMPLICATIONS

You need to consider other possible complications during a rescue. The diver may have an injury or diving malady, such as decompression sickness, a squeeze, air embolism, wound, or heart attack. Because of the three-dimensional nature of scuba diving, the diver could be upside down, twisted, or entangled. Cold and fatigue are also common problems. Cramps from cold water and/or the hard work of swimming add to complications. Stress leading to panic is, of course, a major complication. Another major complication is collapse, which can lead to an obstructed airway and inability to breathe.

Finally, though not actually a complication, but a primary consideration for you should you ever be called upon to be the rescuer, is pacing. In managing a distressed diver it is important not to exhaust yourself so totally that you are no longer of assistance to the diver in need of your help. With appropriate training from your instructor and practice of your rescue skills you will find your "pace." An emergency can then be appropriately managed, leaving you with sufficient reserve to manage the situation when you get the diver in need of care to the boat or shore.

Diving Equipment

Even though some equipment may be in the way or impose some limitations to movement during a rescue, equipment greatly enhances the ease and safety of diving rescues. Equipment makes diver rescues easier and safer than rescuing a non-diving swimmer.

The mask lets you see underwater, protects your face, and enables you to maintain relatively clear vision even when splashed or hit with chop on the surface. Fins give you the power, speed, and maneuverability to reach a victim or get out of a tight situation yourself. Both the snorkel and scuba equipment offer alternate breathing methods. Protection and reserve buoyancy come from the wet suit. The buoyancy compensator (BC) makes resting and mouth-to-mouth resuscitation at the surface reasonable possibilities. Surface floats add another dimension of ease and safety to diving and compasses can be used during diver rescue tows. Diver's knives can be used to cut entanglements or as all-purpose tools. Finally, whistle can be used to call for help.

There are some additional equipment considerations to remember during diver rescues. Any breathing resistance due to diving equipment can add to the work of a diving rescue. You should use the easiest way to breathe in any particular situation. Remember, breathing through your mouth at the surface is the easiest possible way and this method of breathing is also the greatest stress-reducer for the diver in distress. Anything held in your hands, if you are going to initiate a rescue, should either be ditched or passed off to another diver. If you feel that gloves or mitts may be a hindrance, they may have to be removed prior to attempting a rescue. Practice will be the only way to determine in advance what equipment changes will be required during a rescue.

In an emergency situation, when positive buoyancy is necessary, it should be an automatic response to inflate the BC, ditch the weight belt, or both. Weight belts should be easily identifiable on the diver, equipped with an accessible quick-release buckle, and have the buckle oriented opposite the buckle securing the BC. Weights should be ditched vertically with the weight belt held away from the diver's body before being released to prevent entanglement with other equipment. The BC should be equipped with a power inflator.

Rescue Situations and Procedures
SELF-AID

If more divers were truly competent at self-aid there would be significantly fewer incidents of the more dramatic rescues.

Your first line of defense against diving difficulties should be prevention. When prevention has failed and you still have a problem, you should be prepared to deal with difficulties and the accompanying stress by providing self-aid. This is by far the most important and most used form of rescue. Because self-aid is not dramatic and

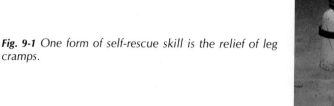

Fig. 9-1 *One form of self-rescue skill is the relief of leg cramps.*

does not require outside help, it most often goes unnoticed. In addition, many everyday diving skills are self-help, and self-assistance techniques. These include:

1. Buoyancy control, with power inflator, oral inflator, or CO_2, as well as low-stress resting on the surface.
2. Emergency swimming and buoyant ascents.
3. Survival swimming techniques, such as treading water, bobbing or drown-proofing, floating, swimming in place, or snorkel breathing.
4. Ditching the weight belt system.
5. Changing to alternate fin kicks when tired, such as flutter, scissors, dolphin, or frog kicks; or swimming on your back.
6. Being able to take-off, adjust, and replace dive gear on the surface.
7. Relieving leg cramps (Fig. 9-1) by stopping activity, holding the fin tip, and straightening or massaging the cramped leg.
8. Switching from one breathing method to another, as needed, such as snorkel, scuba, or with no equipment.
9. Mask and regulator clearing.

Much of your basic diver training taught you to take care of difficulties for yourself, but this clearly does not prevent your buddy from lending you a helping hand. In fact, this is the best way to handle a problem, such as relieving a cramp that has occurred (Fig. 9-2). Your buddy assists by massaging the affected leg. Working together to solve the problem has the added advantage that you are both aware of the problem and can adjust activities to suit the problem.

BUDDY ASSIST

The buddy assist is a natural outgrowth of working together and of the relationship you and your buddy already have. It can be as simple as the reassuring touch of your hand on your buddy's arm or as extensive as towing your buddy all the way to

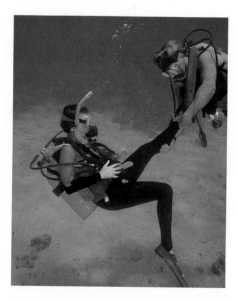

Fig. 9-2 *By having your buddy help in the relief of a leg cramp, you are both aware of the problem. After correcting the immediate difficulty you can adjust the dive plan as needed.*

shore. Quite often, the assist will be so natural that it seems to have no relation to diver rescue. Other times, it will be apparent to both you and your buddy that a situation could have turned into a serious diving accident if one of you had not assisted the other.

Again, during your diver training, you acquired many skills that may be used to help your buddy. These same skills are often used in the more serious situation of the buddy rescue:

1. Helping your buddy hold, remove, and replace gear
2. Inflating your buddy's BC (Fig. 9-3)
3. Towing your buddy
4. Ditching your buddy's equipment, particularly the weight belt (Fig. 9-4)
5. Helping your buddy who is entangled
6. Responding to your buddy's hand signals
7. Sharing air
8. Buddy breathing, since this may be the only available option

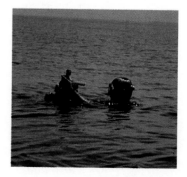

Fig. 9-3 *A buddy, in an emergency, inflates his buddy's BC.*

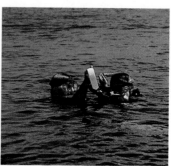

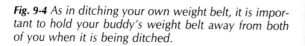

Fig. 9-4 *As in ditching your own weight belt, it is important to hold your buddy's weight belt away from both of you when it is being ditched.*

In the normal course of diving activities, you and your buddy should use and practice these skills. This makes these skills a natural and comfortable part of diving. When your buddy needs assistance, approach so you can be seen, and make both visual and physical contact. The touch of your hand, many times, reassures your buddy. Both of you should then stop, breathe easy, think, communicate, and proceed when you are both under control.

Proceed slowly and easily, as rushing increases the stress level. Be sure to use available equipment to make the assist as easy as possible. If you are on the bottom, solve the problem there if at all possible and check your instruments to gain a more secure sense of orientation.

If you are on the surface, use positive buoyancy to make it easier to solve the problem and be sure to solve the problem and talk over the solution. Have your buddy use the easiest possible way to breathe and, if needed, help your buddy by using a simple tow through the water.

BUDDY RESCUE

The buddy rescue is performed when prevention, self-aid, or a buddy assist has failed or is not appropriate. Rescues are also used when the situation would lead directly and immediately to a serious diving accident, if an outsider did not intervene. These are the most difficult rescues to perform and, fortunately, the least often needed. The panicked diver or the diver who has collapsed into unconsciousness and is not breathing requires this type of rescue. However, remember that self-aid and buddy assists make up the vast majority of all rescues. Diver rescues involving panic or collapse are rare.

The significance of distinguishing between buddy assist and the buddy rescue relates directly to human values. During a buddy assist, neither the victim nor the rescuer is in any great danger. The assist is easy for the rescuer and does not embarrass the victim. However, during a buddy rescue, both the victim and the rescuer are in real danger, particularly the victim. Such a rescue is extremely difficult and requires considerable outside help and support. This rescue will make great demands on your physical resources of skill, strength, and courage. Everyday life does not prepare most people for dealing with such emergencies.

The assist and rescue have similar techniques. Often a rescue becomes an assist as soon as the victim calms down or, sometimes, the diver being assisted ends up needing to be rescued. Most often, you or your buddy perform assists and rescues, but in some cases an instructor, lifeguard, boat crew, or even a passing diver will handle the situation. This may happen because an outside person is better qualified, physically or mentally, to make the rescue, because the buddies are separated, or because both buddies are in trouble.

The rescue primarily uses diving skills you have already learned. These skills do not require great precision, but they do require added urgency because your buddy may have panicked or be unconscious. Most of the additional skills you need in a rescue are common first-aid techniques. Specifically, these skills include:

1. All buddy assist skills
2. Handling a struggling buddy underwater or on the surface
3. Bringing an unconscious buddy to the surface
4. Handling an unconscious buddy on the surface
5. Mouth-to-mouth or mouth-to-mask resuscitation on the surface
6. Cardiopulmonary resuscitation (CPR)
7. Taking care of yourself during a buddy rescue (see comments at the beginning of this chapter relative to pacing)
8. Searching for a missing diver

Struggling and Panic

Your buddy may quickly progress from a state of stress, to struggling, to panic. As soon as you are aware of a problem, move in, evaluate whether or not there is any immediate threat to yourself, and assist your buddy as needed. The effects, signs, and symptoms of stress are your clues to trouble. If your buddy is already struggling or is panicked, you must take care to protect yourself. Think quickly before acting, then take action, leaving yourself a way out if the situation should get out of control.

The worst panic situation is underwater, because your buddy might take your regulator mouthpiece or knock off your mask. Fortunately, you will probably never see a panicked diver underwater. In many underwater panic cases, the diver's survival instinct overpowers proper training and the diver tries to escape to the surface. If you are helping your buddy underwater and the situation does get out of control, push away, and take care of yourself. If this does not work or does not seem reasonable, make your buddy positively buoyant, if at all possible, by ditching his or her weight belt first then inflating the buddy's BC using the power inflator. Next, make yourself positively buoyant. Practice of these skills is of paramount importance in order for you, the potential rescuer, to determine the effect of ditching your weight belt on your ability to effect a rescue. Some divers experience such a dramatic shift in center of gravity on ditching the weight belt that they can no longer function in a practical position relative to the victim once brought to the surface. For most divers, it's probably not a good idea to ditch the weight belt when attempting a rescue on another. Once you as the rescuer have established positive

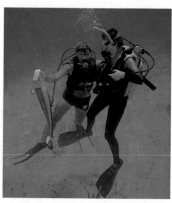

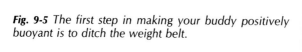

Fig. 9-5 The first step in making your buddy positively buoyant is to ditch the weight belt.

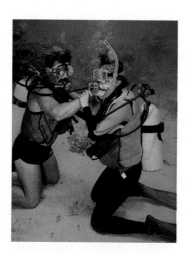

Fig. 9-6 Utilizing the octopus to share air is an effective, less skill-intensive way to share air.

buoyancy, take the buddy to the surface and sort out the situation. These situations make easily accessible, quick-release weight belt buckles, power inflators, and alternate regulators or other source of alternate air *absolutely mandatory* for all scuba divers (Figs. 9-5 through 9-8).

A struggling diver on the surface is still dangerous, but you have more options for rescue. Again, stop and think before acting. If your buddy is struggling and has not yet panicked, or you see the cause of the difficulty and believe you can immediately help, establish verbal and eye contact with your buddy, then immediately move in and act. Your physical contact and action may stop the evolution of the situation toward panic and bring the situation under control. Whenever possible, use positive buoyancy for your own protection and establish positive buoyancy for your buddy as rapidly as possible, if the buddy is not already positively buoyant (Fig. 9-9).

If the situation is more desperate and you are unsure you can be effective or safe when reaching your buddy, approach from where your buddy can see you;

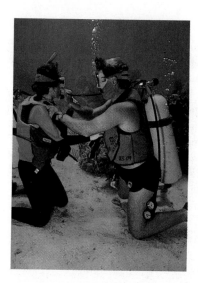

Fig. 9-7 *Buddy breathing from a single second stage is the least desirable way to share air but is a skill that regular buddies should practice so it can be performed in an emergency.*

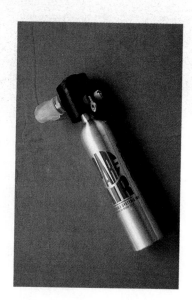

Fig. 9-8 *This is one of several options that might be employed as an alternate source of air to be utilized in an emergency should your primary source be lost. However, such air supplies are quite limited and should provide only the brief supply necessary to effect a safe, immediate ascent.*

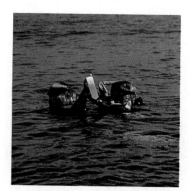

Fig. 9-9 *If contact is made with your buddy, you should quickly make the buddy positively buoyant by first ditching the weight belt.*

stop, and shout clear but brief and simple instructions. Try to make your buddy relax and take action. If your buddy swims toward you, simply back up toward the safety of the boat or shore (Fig. 9-10). While you are dealing with your buddy, you should also be trying to alert diving companions on the shore or the crew of the boat that you are involved in an emergency situation and may require assistance.

If you feel that a rescue attempt is required, one method is to grab your buddy's arm (your right arm grasping buddy's right arm or your left arm grasping your buddy's left arm) and rapidly pull, while spinning your buddy toward you. This action will pull your buddy toward you and spin your buddy so his or her back and tank will be facing you. You can gain control of your buddy by grasping the tank valve with your right hand and squeezing the buddy's tank between your knees. This leaves your left hand available to reach over the buddy's left shoulder and use the power inflator on the buddy's BC to add buoyancy. Often, getting the buddy under control and establishing the buddy's buoyancy will defuse a serious situation. Figs. 9-11 through 9-14 illustrate the steps in this type of buddy rescue.

If your buddy does grab you during the rescue attempt and you are in distress, first attempt to break away by pushing off with your hand or foot. If that is not suc-

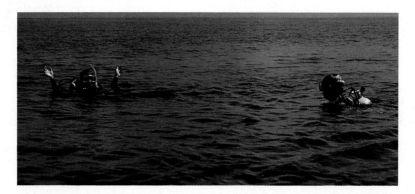

Fig. 9-10 *The approach to the buddy at the surface should maintain sufficient distance between you and your buddy.*

Fig. 9-11 *The buddy's arm is grasped and you spin and pull the buddy towards you.*

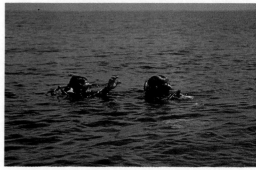

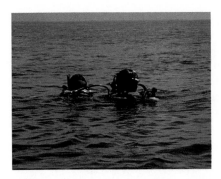

Fig. 9-12 The buddy will come toward you with the tank facing you. Prevent your buddy from grabbing you if panic sets in.

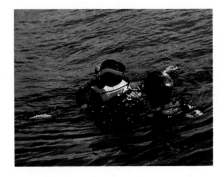

Fig. 9-13 Control of the buddy is maintained by grasping the tank valve in the right hand and squeezing the buddy's tank between your knees. You have control over the buddy, remain clear of the buddy's grasp, and bring him or her back into a position where the face is out of the water, a position that should put him or her more at ease. This is called a tank-cradle technique of rescue.

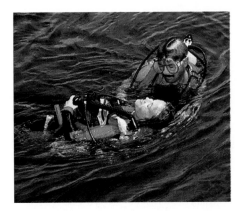

Fig. 9-14 If wave conditions permit, the buddy may be put more at ease after the buoyancy is established by removing the mask and exposing the face to the fresh air. If wave action is rough, the mask should be left in place.

cessful, then you should go underwater, as this is the last place that your panicked buddy will want to follow you. Situations such as this should not develop if your approach is cautious or you utilize the method shown above for gaining control. Remember, establishing positive buoyancy is paramount, first for your buddy then for you. If someone from the shore or the boat can get a surface float to you, give that to the buddy as well, or perhaps this could be the first step in getting the buddy under control if the float is readily available.

During panic, divers cannot help themselves, but if you wait until your buddy collapses from struggling, then you may have to deal with a drowning or heart attack. If your talking, actions, or other methods discussed thus far either do not work or you do not feel comfortable with them, and the panic persists, then an underwater approach may be appropriate. Go onto scuba and descend. Approach your buddy from underneath and behind. First, ditch the buddy's weight belt from under the water but stay behind the buddy to avoid being kicked. Then, use the tank-cradle technique shown above to gain control of the buddy for a sufficient period of time to get the BC inflated. With buoyancy established in this manner, you can either continue control as above or simply back off until the buddy calms down with buoyancy established. All of these actions are simply taken without discussion with your buddy since when you reach this point, action is paramount and little will be gained from additional attempts at conversation.

When your buddy is no longer struggling, you can proceed with other necessary assistance, such as towing to safety. Do not concern yourself with the fine details or skillful form during a rescue. Just get your buddy safely buoyant at the surface while keeping yourself from injury and then terminate the dive.

Unconscious Diver

The most serious situation you will ever face is when your buddy is unconscious. In the water, unconsciousness is most frequently accompanied by lack of breathing. Speed is critical in this situation. You must immediately bring your buddy to the surface, open the airway, and start mouth-to-mouth or mouth-to-mask ventilation, if breathing does not start on its own. Then, you must begin to move to the nearest exit point from the water.

It is very unlikely that your buddy will become unconscious and stop breathing while you are diving side-by-side underwater, so this reinforces the need for close contact while diving. It is more likely that you may find your buddy on the bottom and unconscious after you have become separated. Approach and hold your buddy as quickly as possible (Figs. 9-15 and 9-16). If your buddy is entangled or gear is in the way, remove any and all obstructions. You have no way to reasonably control your unconscious buddy's exhalation during ascent, but your buddy will die without air. So, speed to the surface is a must. Immediately establish positive buoyancy for your buddy, hold him or her from the rear or side, if you are on the bottom push off, and swim for the surface (Fig. 9-17). If you feel that you are working too hard during the ascent, then inflate your BC and, as a last resort, consider ditching your weight belt.

If you lose control during the ascent and feel you are ascending too rapidly, place your victim into an attitude of maximum flare to present the greatest surface area to the water to slow the ascent. Be certain to monitor your breathing and be sure that you never hold your breath. If you find yourself struggling to maintain control of the victim and or your ascent, reposition the victim. Some rescue sources recommend letting your victim go but there is the concern that doing so may lead to accusations of abandonment of the victim. That risk needs to be weighed against the risk to your personal safety, which should always be your primary concern.

During the ascent, it may be helpful to tilt your buddy's head back to open the airway since the tongue and epiglottis may be the only obstruction to the blocked

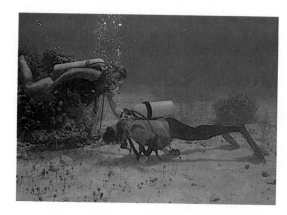

Fig. 9-15 The diver makes contact with his unconscious buddy.

Fig. 9-16 The buddy is turned over, and the rescuing diver quickly gains control of the situation.

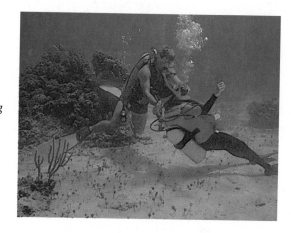

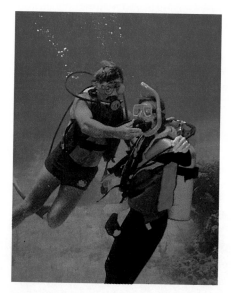

Fig. 9-17 The diver quickly pushes off from the bottom after positive buoyancy has been established or at the same time buoyancy is being established. The rescuer also tries to maintain an open airway and secures the regulator in the unconscious buddy's mouth.

airway and repositioning might possibly stimulate spontaneous breathing. However, the idea that pulmonary over-pressure injuries may occur from improper airway position on ascent does not have significant viability since the natural anatomic direction of airflow is outward, even with a bad airway position. However, these are fine details of technique that are not of proven value. Getting to the surface *immediately* is of proven value.

Once on the surface, float your buddy on his or her back and tilt the head back to open the airway. If the buddy is brought to the surface face-down, you will have to roll the buddy over before taking this step. Spontaneous breathing often starts when the airway is opened. If breathing does not immediately start and there is a pulse, which you can check at the carotid artery while opening the airway, start mouth-to-mask or mouth-to-mouth resuscitation. If a pulse is not present, continue artificial ventilation while moving as quickly as possible to an exit point where CPR can be performed.

Missing Diver

Someday, your buddy or some other diver in your group may be missing. It is human nature to want to take immediate action and have every available diver enter the water for the search. This is both dangerous and an ineffective way to find the missing diver. As with most other diving emergencies, stop, think, and get control, then take action. First, get answers to several vital questions. Who is with the missing diver? Where was the missing diver last seen? When did the dive start and when was the diver missed? How much air did the missing diver have? What kind of equipment was the missing diver using and what are the dominant colors of this equipment? Did the missing diver have any known difficulties? Who is available, equipped, and qualified to search for the missing diver?

Hopefully, the dive is being done from a dive boat with an underwater sound recall system; this should be used before any search is begun. The search plan should use only qualified divers who have the experience and equipment and no decompression problems. Buddy pairs start the search and might utilize some of the patterns described in Chapter 6, in the area where the diver was last seen. A safety diver with a surface float should be stationed on the surface and someone on the surface or shore should be in overall charge of the search operation. During the search, other details can be arranged, such as special equipment, communications, and transportation.

If the search is not successful in a short time, the plan should be changed and local authorities advised. It is very important to notify local authorities as soon as possible that a lost diver situation has arisen. Your ongoing efforts need not be interfered with by notifying local authorities. Instead, such notification should simply be a part of your accident management plan. How long the search lasts is determined by how much air was in the missing diver's tank or weather and light conditions. As with all other rescue situations, safety of the rescuers remains a primary consideration.

It is possible that you may be the only other person involved and your buddy is missing. In this case, you have all the necessary information. You are limited by your own resources of experience, equipment, skill, endurance, and air supply. Do not risk your own safety in a poorly organized search, but do what you can. If you are not successful, get help and notify the proper authorities.

Helicopter Evacuation

Serious boating or diving accidents sometimes require that the injured person be evacuated by helicopter. This is usually done by the U.S. Coast Guard in the United States or the Canadian Coast Guard in Canada, but military or police helicopters may also perform rescues. When you suspect that critical medical care is needed, contact the Coast Guard as soon as possible. Follow their instructions. Use the radio frequency 2182 kHz or VHF channel 16 (156.800 mHz), or other frequencies specified by the Coast Guard or authorities in the area where you may be diving. Continuously listen to the radio for further instructions after you have made the initial contact.

Most rescue helicopters will be able to contact you on a radio frequency compatible with the equipment on board your diving boat. Advise the helicopter, to the best of your ability, of your location before it arrives so the pilot can make a proper approach. Display a distress signal on the boat so the helicopter knows which boat has requested help.

Select and clear the most suitable hoist area on the deck, which will probably be at the stern. Clearing a deck means to remove anything that might become airborne in a strong wind—such items can be very injurious in a helicopter propwash. If the boat has no clear deck area, it may be necessary to tow a dingy or raft behind. If the hoist is at night, light the area as well as possible. Be sure you do not shine any lights on the helicopter as you may blind the pilot. If there are obstructions in the vicinity, advise the pilot of them and put a light on them so the pilot can see them.

Next, secure all loose gear and remove any antennas or poles that might be in the way. Be sure you can still communicate on the radio after you remove the antennas. There will be a high noise level under the helicopter, so conversation between the deck crew will be almost impossible. Change course and speed as directed by the pilot, which will probably involve turning into the wind.

If you do not have radio contact with the helicopter, signal a "come on" when you are in all respects ready for the hoist. Commonly accepted hand signals should be acceptable but the ideal is to have another craft with radio communication capability stand-by to communicate with the helicopter for you. Use a flashlight at night. Allow the basket or stretcher to touch down on the deck prior to handling to avoid static shock. If a trail line is dropped by the helicopter, guide the basket or stretcher to the deck with the line. The line will not cause shock.

Place the person in the basket sitting with hands clear of the sides or strap the person into the stretcher. Place a PFD on the person if possible. Signal the helicopter hoist operator when ready for hoist. The person in the basket or stretcher should nod if possible. Deck personnel then give the "thumbs-up" signal.

If it is necessary to take the stretcher away from the hoist point, unhook the cable and keep it free for the helicopter to haul in the hoist cable. *Do not hook the cable to the vessel or attempt to move the stretcher or basket without unhooking it.*

When the person is strapped in the stretcher or basket, signal the helicopter to lower the cable, hook up again, and signal the hoist operator when ready to hoist. Keep the stretcher from swinging or turning. If a trail line is attached to the stretcher or basket, use it to steady. Be sure to send complete information with the victim of a diving accident.

Rescue Skills

A book simply can in no way teach you the vital skills involved in rescue but can only serve as a guide for skills to be taught by a professional instructor. Many agencies offer training in lifesaving, CPR, first-aid, and swimming. These courses help to prepare you to handle emergencies (Fig. 9-18). However, these courses do not fully prepare you to handle scuba-related emergencies. All major scuba training agencies offer courses in rescue, and in recent years several courses have been developed to appropriately train scuba divers in the management of emergencies that may occur in the scuba environment. Consult with your local professionally managed dive store for referrals to such specialized courses.

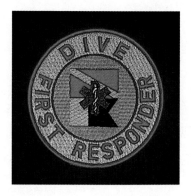

Fig. 9-18 *Courses are available to supplement rescue training so that you will be comfortable with the management of the rescued diver in an emergency.*

Tows

Tows include various techniques for moving a diver who needs help through the water to a safer place, either boat or shore. While towing, you become aware of environmental and other complications that make rescues difficult. Several important principles make diving tows more effective:

1. The rescuer moves slowly and paces progress to prevent exhaustion during the assist.
2. Contact and control is maintained by the rescuer.
3. The buddy being towed is in a position permitting easy breathing.
4. The buddy being towed is positively buoyant and has had unnecessary gear, especially the weight belt, ditched. The rescuer, as well, should be positively buoyant as needed for comfort and ease of swimming.

5. The buddy being towed is maintained in as nearly a horizontal position as possible. This makes towing easier as the horizontal body position presents the least amount of resistance.
6. The buddy being towed is in a position where he or she is free to swim and "assist with the assist." If possible, the buddy can do an easy fin kick to help.
7. The rescuer is in a safe position so contact with the buddy can be terminated if necessary, should the situation deteriorate into a full-blown rescue.
8. If someone is there who can assist you, take advantage of their help. If artificial ventilation is required, one can tow while the other maintains the victim's breathing.
9. Change positions as needed to avoid specific muscle group fatigue problems and cramping.

Tows do not require the graceful techniques of synchronized swimming, so fine details of technique are not of primary consideration. Tows are crude but effective ways to help another diver. By remembering the principles above and trying the following techniques, you can do anything to get the job done. Most divers find certain techniques and positions work better than others. Still, the details are left up to you—whatever works!

Towing beside your buddy (Fig. 9-19) is the position used most often. Sometimes called the do-si-do because of the interlocked arms, similar to square dancers, the position allows you to maintain control of your buddy by holding onto the BC, tank valve, wet suit, or anything that's easy to get your hand on. Without interlocking arms, you can simply place your hand into the buddy's armpit. This tow is the best position for closely monitoring your buddy or performing artificial ventilation if needed. It also allows you to easily talk with your buddy, sometimes a very calming influence in a stressful situation.

Tows from the buddy's head are utilized when the buddy is conscious, breathing, and relatively comfortable. These tows are sometimes faster and easier to perform than others but they do not give the same close physical contact and directional control of other tows. You may hold onto your buddy with one hand on the BC, tank valve, wet suit neck, a strap, or the buddy's chin. You can hold the bud-

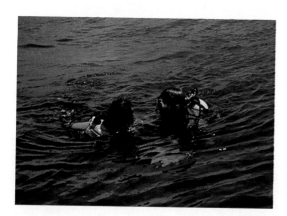

Fig. 9-19 *The do-si-do assist is used when you want to tow your buddy but also want to be as close as possible to monitor your buddy's condition.*

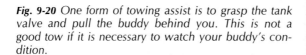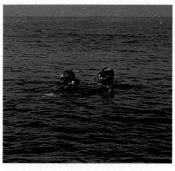

Fig. 9-20 One form of towing assist is to grasp the tank valve and pull the buddy behind you. This is not a good tow if it is necessary to watch your buddy's condition.

dy's head with both hands if necessary. This maintains physical contact with your buddy and may provide a calming influence. When towing by any of your buddy's equipment, be certain that your action does not interfere with your buddy's breathing (Fig. 9-20).

A third form of tow is really a push. Usually reserved for tired but calm and stable divers, the technique involves the buddy laying horizontally with his or her fins resting on your shoulders. The tired diver should maintain his or her legs in an outstretched position, spread apart, and you can put your hands on top of the tired diver's legs while you swim pushing. Another version of this same technique is to have the tired swimmer place his or her hands on your shoulders with the push being performed in the same manner. The advantage of these techniques is the ability to see where you are going. Though it is highly unlikely for the positively buoyant victim to panic, if that is a concern in your mind then having your head between the victim's legs would probably not be ideal, so you might wish to push with your hands on the fins instead of your shoulders. This would enable you to break contact with a panicked diver more quickly (Fig. 9-21).

All of the tows described involve the buddy floating face-up. However, if you are towing the tired diver using a surface float, your buddy could lie face down and breathe through the regulator or snorkel. These are very easy tows for tired divers.

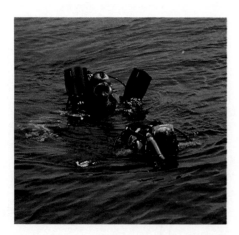

Fig. 9-21 You can assist your buddy in need of a "tow" by employing the fin push.

When two divers are available to make a rescue, one should be at the victim's side for artificial ventilation, if needed, or to reassure the conscious diver. The second rescuer should be positioned at victim's head for towing. When there are three divers doing the rescue, one remains at the victim's head for towing, while the other two are at the victim's sides for towing, ditching gear, artificial ventilation, or reassurance while continuing to tow. By using your compass while towing, you do not have to watch your destination; you can watch your buddy while still maintaining directional control.

Leaving the Water

If your buddy can still function, exiting the water simply involves assisting the buddy to remove gear and get out of the water at the end of the rescue. If your buddy cannot help then enlist any bystander's aid.

When removing your buddy from the water, remove all equipment that will not be necessary so the victim is the only thing that needs to be managed without the excess weight. In a full-blown rescue, you can gradually ditch the victim's unnecessary gear starting with the weight belt, as you move toward the boat or shore; scuba tank, mask, and any other negatively buoyant equipment attached to the victim should be dumped. Depending upon the rescue conditions, you may not wish to dump the victim's mask but, instead, loop its strap around your arm. Though mask removal aids in artificial ventilation during the rescue, it may be useful to afford the injured diver some protection during the exit, particularly in the surf. So reapplying the mask to the victim's face prior to exit may be appropriate.

If diving alone with your buddy from a small boat, exit from the water is more difficult. After removing all possible equipment from your buddy, place both of the buddy's hands on the boat gunwale (Fig. 9-22). Be sure his or her face is above water. Now, while holding your buddy's hands with one of yours, give a strong kick with your fins and climb in the boat while continuing to hold the buddy's hands with one of yours. Next, grab your buddy's wrists and pull or drag your buddy over the gunwale to the waist, then roll the buddy the rest of the way into the boat. This

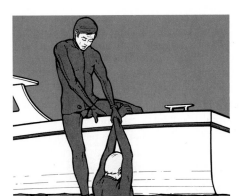

Fig. 9-22 Removing the buddy from the water.

may work in a small boat such as an inflatable. If you are in the practice of diving with only your buddy from a small boat, you should both develop an emergency method for getting each other back into the boat and practice it regularly so you will not have to "experiment" in a time of emergency.

If your rescue goes to the shore, rather than to a boat, ditch maximum gear before reaching shore and obtain bystander help if possible. If you are alone with the victim, drag or pull the victim from the water any way possible. Sometimes, you may accomplish this by putting your hands through his or her armpits and dragging the victim. Another method, is to spin the victim around by his or her feet, after clear of the water and drag the victim up the beach using the ankles as grips. If you are on a beach and CPR will be necessary or you are dealing with an unconscious diving accident victim, you want the victim placed with their head down on the slope of the beach.

Artificial Ventilation

Under Cardiopulmonary Resuscitation, which follows, you will learn the detailed steps of the procedure for artificial ventilation. Providing artificial ventilation in the water is an adaptation of the standard method. There are, however, two special techniques that can be employed in the water to manage the non-breathing victim.

MOUTH-TO-MOUTH/MOUTH-TO-MASK VENTILATION

The first technique is an adaptation of the technique used on land. The victim's nose is pinched off or occluded with the nose pocket of the diving mask and ventilation takes place using the mouth-to-mouth technique. With the fear of infection today, however, mouth-to-mask is preferable and there are masks on the market today that can be used with one hand and still maintain an adequate seal and permit effective ventilation of the victim. This technique requires a great deal of practice to gain competence and you cannot depend upon the pocket mask to maintain the seal. Instead, in addition to ventilation, you must be certain the seal is maintained and your nonbreathing diver is actually being ventilated with each breath administered. The ideal way to perform either of these skills would probably be with the diving mask removed, but with adequate practice you can do it effectively either way (Fig. 9-23).

MOUTH-TO-SNORKEL VENTILATION

An emergency ventilation technique that was popularized in the 1970s is mouth-to-snorkel ventilation. With one hand under the victim's chin, you maintain control of the victim's airway, apply pressure upward to seal off the nose with the mask nose-pocket, keep the victim's snorkel in place, and maintain contact necessary to tow the victim through the water. The other hand is used to hold the snorkel to the rescuer's mouth so ventilations can be given down the snorkel barrel. When initially developed, this was an excellent rescue technique for snorkelers in distress, but today most snorkels sold have purge valves that make this method of resuscitation impossible (Fig. 9-24).

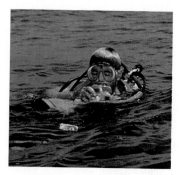

Fig. 9-23 *Mouth-to-mask ventilation can be performed while you are towing the victim to an appropriate exit point.*

Fig. 9-24 *Mouth-to-snorkel ventilation may be useful when wave conditions might make it inappropriate to use mouth-to-mask or mouth-to-mouth ventilation. With most modern snorkels being equipped with purge valves, this technique will usually not work and the victim should be quickly taken to the nearest appropriate exit point.*

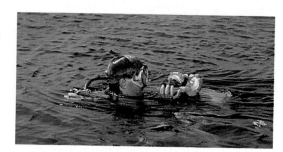

In-Water Rescue Procedures

During the actual rescue process, you need to be guided by your capabilities and what, at the moment, appears to hold the best prospect for your victim's ultimate survival. There are various schools of thought regarding what the rescuer should do in the way of resuscitation in water. The extremes range from in-water CPR when the rescuer has the victim a long distance from shore or the rescue boat to the other extreme, which advocates simply getting the victim to the boat or shore.

Appropriate victim care will be largely dictated by circumstances. If the rescue itself will be arduous and no additional help is available, the rescuer has to consider conservation of energy so that proper CPR can be performed on the victim upon reaching the boat or shore. In some cases, the apparently dead diver may be stimulated to breathe spontaneously with the initiation of mouth-to-mask ventilation. A diver who keeps a pocket mask as an essential piece of equipment accompanying the BC can administer rescue breaths to the victim immediately upon getting the victim to the surface if water conditions are not so rough to present a risk to the victim's airway. It is reasonable to assume that artificial ventilation can only be performed in a marginal fashion while towing the victim through the water and that in-water CPR is of little value. With that in mind, it probably makes more sense to try to ventilate the victim upon surfacing in an effort to trigger spontaneous breathing. If that is unsuccessful then the rescuer's priority should probably be to get the victim to a location, shore or boat, where proper CPR can be performed. If water conditions permit and the rescuer determines that the victim has a pulse or makes that assumption, then ventilations of 1.5 to 2.0 seconds each should be delivered to the victim every 5 seconds during the rescue. As with any rescues, if the rescuer decides that attempting to ventilate the victim may place the rescuer himself or herself at risk, then the objective should be to get the victim to the boat or shore.

Cardiopulmonary Resuscitation

Though this skill is often divided into mouth-to-mouth resuscitation and CPR, the entire process is actually a continuum. The procedure that will be described is how the victim should be attended to whether or not both breathing and heartbeat have stopped or only breathing has stopped. In addition, as we will discuss below, the process can be started in the water.

Though the material here is quite thorough, you should seek out specialized training in cardiopulmonary resuscitation from the American Heart Association, The American National Red Cross, or the equivalent organization in your country if you are not being trained in the United States.

The purpose of cardiopulmonary resuscitation is to supply the victim's body with oxygen and, if necessary, maintain the victim's circulation until normal breathing resumes. You may be called upon to perform this level of care until emergency medical services personnel can relieve you or until you are no longer physically capable of continuing (Figs. 9-25 through 9-33). Cardiopulmonary resuscitation should be continued until the victim begins to breath spontaneously, you are too weak to continue, you are relieved by someone else who knows how to do cardiopulmonary resuscitation, or until the victim is placed in the hands of emergency medical services personnel.

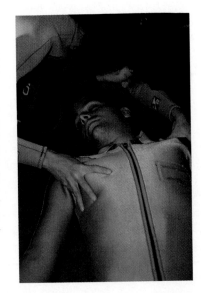

Fig. 9-25 The first step is to determine whether or not the victim has simply fainted. If the individual is not already on his or her back, you will have to roll him or her over into a face-up position on a firm surface. The deck of a boat or pool or the firm sand of a beach are OK. This can be accomplished by gently shaking the victim and shouting near his or her ear, "Hey, are you OK?" or something like that. If the victim does not respond or regain consciousness, it is necessary for you to continue in the process as well as having other people on the boat or at the beach or pool begin the process of mobilizing whatever emergency medical service assistance is available. If a diver has simply fainted, he or she will usually regain consciousness immediately or soon after lying down.

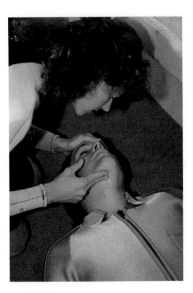

Fig. **9-26** *If the diver did not respond, you must next open the victim's airway. This is accomplished by what is called the head-tilt, chin-lift method. The hand toward the top of the victim's head is placed on the victim's forehead while two or three fingers are placed under the victim's jaw as shown. By lifting with the fingers under the jaw and, at the same time, pressing down and back on the victim's forehead, the head is rotated back in what is called a hyperextended position. This will lift the tongue and other structures that might be blocking the airway of the patient. Sometimes, it may only be necessary to perform this procedure to stimulate the victim to breathe on his or her own.*

Fig. **9-27** *Now, lean your head down over the victim's face as shown and maintain this position for between 3 to 5 seconds. Keep your ear near the victim's nose and mouth, and watch the victim's chest. You are looking for the rise and fall of the victim's chest while trying to breathe and listening and feeling for the movement of air in and out of the victim's mouth and nose.*

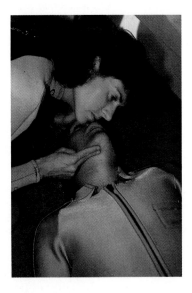

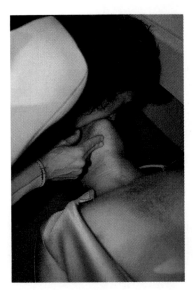

Fig. **9-28** *If the victim is not breathing, you must initiate mouth-to-mouth breathing for the victim (mouth-to-mask is probably safer if you are concerned with the risk of infection). This is done by pinching the victim's nostrils closed with the hand you already have on the victim's forehead. Then cover the victim's mouth with your own and give two full ventilations, or rescue breaths, to the victim. These breaths should be slow, full ventilations taking 1½ to 2 seconds per breath. Between these breaths, allow the victim to exhale passively.*

Fig. 9-29 *After giving the two rescue breaths as above, it is necessary to check the victim's pulse to learn if the heart is still beating. This procedure is done by sliding two finger tips into the indentation next to the trachea in the groove-like indentation between the trachea and the major muscle running down the side of the neck. In this indentation, you will be able to feel pulsations of the heart through the carotid artery if the heart is still beating. You should take 5 to 10 seconds to take the victim's pulse before going any further. If you feel a pulse, then the victim's heart is still beating, and you need to go no further in the CPR process. However, if the victim is still not breathing, then you will have to give the victim rescue breaths at a rate of one breath every 5 seconds (12 breaths per minute). You should also recheck the pulse every few minutes to be certain the victim's heart is still beating. This rescue breathing must continue until the victim begins to breathe on his or her own or until you are relieved.*

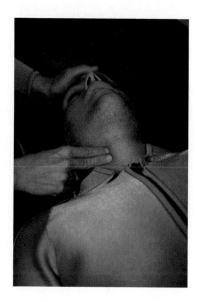

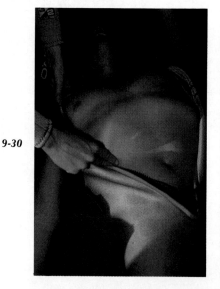

9-30

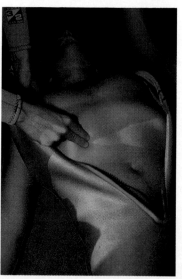

9-31

Figs. 9-30 and 9-31 *If you determine that the patient is pulseless, then the heart is not beating. You will then have to initiate chest compressions along with rescue breathing that has already been started. Expose the victim's chest if it is not already bared. Take two finger-tips from your hand closest to the victim's feet and draw those finger tips along the lower border of the victim's rib cage until you come to the bottom of the victim's sternum (breastbone). Leave those two fingers where they are now resting (your fingers now rest on the xiphoid process, or lowest segment of the sternum) and place your hand that is closest to the patient's head on the sternum immediately above your two fingers remaining in place.*

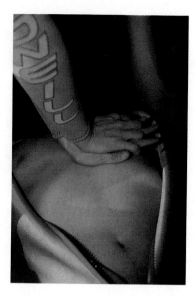

Fig. 9-32 *Now place the hand that is closest to the victim's feet on top of the hand already resting on the sternum and begin to compress the sternum at a rate of 80 to 100 times per minute. Each stroke with the two hands on the chest should compress the chest at least 1½ inches but not more than 2 inches. After compressing the victim's chest for 15 compressions, ventilate the victim two more times as described in Fig. 9-28. This alternating of 15 chest compressions with two ventilations should continue. After four cycles of compressions and ventilations, recheck the pulse exactly in the same manner as described in Fig. 9-29. If the pulse has returned, then continue rescue breathing as needed. If there has been no return of pulse, ventilate the patient twice, as in Fig. 9-28, and continue the chest compressions and ventilations at the same rate as above.*

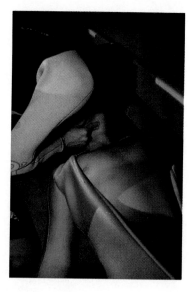

Fig. 9-33 *Here the rescuer gives the victim the two ventilations, which are given between every 15 compressions.*

First Aid

First aid is the "immediate and temporary care of an injured person." First aid is not medical care but temporary care until the injured party can be transferred to appropriate emergency medical care or definitive medical care.

Some form of first aid training is useful for divers and it would be appropriate for you to seek out training that might be helpful in an emergency. Well prepared

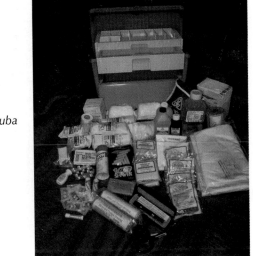

Fig. 9-34 The first aid kit of the well-prepared scuba diver.

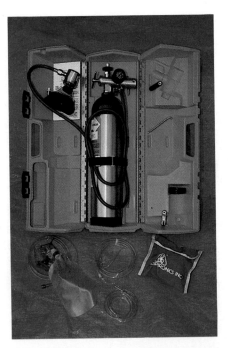

Fig. 9-35 Responsible divers and dive operators should carry an oxygen unit equipped with a positive pressure demand valve unit for administering 100% oxygen to injured divers.

divers also carry a well-equipped first aid kit with them while diving (Fig. 9-34) and more and more divers are carrying oxygen with them similar to the unit shown in Fig. 9-35.

As with all diving emergencies, stop and think. Do what you can, but be careful not to cause any further injury. If you know what to do and are dealing with a diving injury, proceed with the care appropriate for diving accidents.

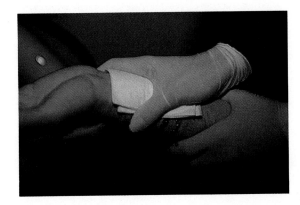

Fig. 9-36 *Direct pressure and elevation is typically all that is required to stop severe bleeding. The wound should then be covered with a dry sterile dressing, and the injured diver should be taken for medical care.*

The most serious accidents in diving are a result of pressure changes encountered in diving, such as decompression sickness, air embolism, and other lung overpressure accidents. The first aid for these is the same:

1. Keep the victim lying down on his or her back, keeping the victim flat.
2. Initiate cardiopulmonary resuscitation if needed.
3. Continuously administer oxygen by the method that will deliver the highest concentration to the victim.
4. Treat the victim for shock, primarily by preventing any further heat loss.
5. Mobilize the local emergency medical services system—in many parts of the United States this can be done by phone by dialing "911."
6. Have the victim transported to the nearest facility with an available recompression chamber. If unknown, call Divers Alert Network (DAN) at (919) 684-8111 collect.

WOUNDS

Cuts and scrapes are probably the most common of all diving injuries. Treatment is aimed at stopping bleeding and preventing infection. Small wounds can be managed by washing with soap and water and covering with a sterile dressing. Maintaining cleanliness is the most significant aspect of continuing treatment for small wounds.

Serious bleeding can best be managed by direct pressure to the wound and elevation if the wound is on an extremity (Fig. 9-36). With today's risk of infection, first aid kits should contain gloves to protect the giver of first aid from contact with blood or other bodily fluids. With more advanced first aid training, you may learn about pressure points and tourniquets, but these are rarely needed. Direct pressure should stop most bleeding within 5 to 10 minutes.

SHOCK

Shock is a complex deterioration of many bodily functions that often occurs after serious injury or as a result of some other problem that may be medical or allergic in origin.

All first aid for shock is consistent with the management of any other diving injuries:

1. Keep the victim lying on his or her back. Keep the victim flat unless they are more comfortable in some other position.
2. Calm and reassure the victim as best you can.
3. Keep the victim warm enough to prevent any additional loss of body heat. Do not overheat the victim but prevent further heat loss.
4. Give first aid for any other injuries for which you are able.
5. Administer supplemental oxygen at the highest concentration possible.
6. Be ready to perform artificial ventilation or CPR if required.
7. Do not leave the victim alone.
8. Get emergency medical help.
9. Arrange to transport the victim to medical care as soon as possible.

With the use of oxygen equipment it is best for you to secure the necessary supplemental training. Several programs are available that will teach you how to use the equipment and how to administer oxygen to diving accident victims.

OTHER POSSIBLE FIRST AID PROBLEMS

Marine life envenomations may occur in ocean diving. Most are a result of nematocyst penetrations (stings) from creatures like jellyfish, Portuguese Man-O-War, fire coral, and so forth. Treatment is directed at rinsing the affected area with sea water or sterile saline *(not fresh water)*, removal of any visible tentacles, and pouring white vinegar or diluted household ammonia over the area. Finally, since heat will break down most marine venoms, apply heat to marine envenomations. The temperature should be about the most the injured diver can tolerate. A useful device is the chemical hot pack, which can be carried in first aid kits, triggered when needed, and recycled by boiling after use (Fig. 9-37).

Fractures, strains, and sprains are not usually diving related but more often occur trying to reach the dive site or on the deck of the dive boat. First aid care is directed at immobilization. Joints above and below the suspected injury should be

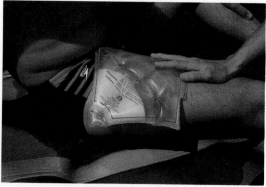

Fig. 9-37 After appropriate initial care, apply heat to marine life envenomations to deactivate the toxins.

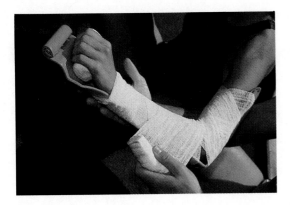

Fig. 9-38 *Treatment of sprains, strains, and fractures is directed at splinting the injury and the joints above and below the location of the suspected injury.*

stabilized, the victim should be treated for shock as needed, and then the victim should be taken to a medical care facility (Fig. 9-38).

Excessive heat can become a truly life-threatening problem. Prevention is the way to deal with heat-related illnesses. Do not allow divers to remain in their gear above water when it's too hot. If divers become overheated to the point where they are hot to the touch, are red in color, stop sweating, and begin to behave in an abnormal manner, this is a true emergency. First aid is directed at getting their body temperature down *fast!* Remove all clothing and dive equipment and keep them drenched with cool water. Keep them out of the sun or remove them from the sun. As quickly as possible, get the victim to a medical facility.

Sunburn is a real problem and it too is usually a matter of prevention. Keep yourself protected from the sun and use liberal amounts of sunscreen. Several commercial preparations are available that will make you or your buddy more comfortable if excessively sunburned.

Seasickness is a problem that was addressed in Chapter 5, and you might wish to take a few moments and glance back at the comments regarding this problem.

External and middle ear problems are often associated with diving. Middle ear problems are usually related to equalization difficulties and typically require that the diver not dive until the problem clears. External ear infections usually require the diver to stop diving as well until the infection is cleared. Prevention of external ear problems amounts to keeping the external ear clean and dry following diving. Several very good commercial preparations are available through your pharmacist to minimize the risk of external ear problems following diving.

Mere knowledge of rescue techniques is not enough to ensure that you will be able to help a diver in a real-life situation. Training and repeated practice can increase both your physical and mental ability to make rescues. It is best to practice in open water rather than pools, so you will be more familiar and comfortable with the environmental conditions. Hopefully, you will never encounter a circumstance requiring diver rescue, but with the combination of proper knowledge, training, and skill, you will be prepared to do anything from simply assisting your buddy to saving a life.

Deep Diving

As you become a more experienced diver, you may wish to expand your horizons and range of qualifications. One area of possible interest and increased diving activity may be dives into deeper water. Deep diving may provide opportunities for the qualified diver that are unavailable at shallower depths. These include shipwrecks, deep reef and rock formations, and drop offs.

Certifying agencies generally limit training for entry-level scuba divers to 60 feet of water or shallower. This, therefore, can be considered as the limit for shallow water diving. Once certified, divers should continue to gain experience while diving within the limits of their training and qualifications. Sixty feet may be viewed as a good depth limit for the novice and inexperienced diver. Diving beyond 130 feet is not recommended for recreational diving. So, we can view shallow diving as depths of from 0 to 60 feet and deep diving beyond 60 feet but not greater than 130 feet.

Dives beyond 130 feet involve increased risk without a proportional increase in benefit and are better left to paid professional divers. Diving beyond 130 feet requires extreme caution, a high degree of training and experience, with particular attention to the effects of nitrogen narcosis, primary and auxiliary air supplies, possible staged decompression, and extensive surface support.

Once certified, divers need to make decisions concerning the limits for their diving experiences. These decisions are borne of knowledge, extent of training, previous experiences, and current qualifications. Some reasons for not diving deeper include increased air consumption, limited bottom time, extended decompression obligation, potential need for staged decompression, and the effects of nitrogen narcosis.

With all the sensible reasons for not diving deep, why do experienced divers still regularly make deep dives? The reasons often include the same feelings generally experienced by all divers including the challenge, adventure, opportunity to explore, an interest in the environment, and often because the goal of the dive just happens to be in deeper water.

After your first scuba diving course, you should seek out other diving courses to gain additional understanding and experience under instructor supervision. These courses will carry such names such as "advanced open water diver," "open water II," "advanced diver," "specialty diver," and other similar names (Fig. 10-1).

It is extremely important to gradually build your experience prior to deep div-

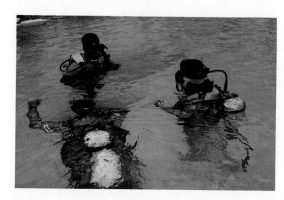

Fig. 10-1 Additional training is necessary before embarking on any deep diving adventures and is a good idea if you have been away from diving for awhile.

ing. This includes slowly increasing your range of skills, activities, and depth. If you stop diving for awhile, you need to decrease your diving depth and then gradually increase depth again. How often you dive may have some effect on how susceptible you will be to nitrogen narcosis and decompression sickness.

Definitions of deep diving and recommendations on diving limits will vary with water conditions and geographic location. A dive, for example, to 60 feet in 40 degree water with only 15 foot visibility in a quarry may require as much or more preparation and experience as a 100 foot dive in warm Caribbean water with 150 foot visibility.

As a diver, you have a responsibility to yourself, your buddy, and the diving community. In order to meet this responsibility, you should understand your personal qualifications and limitations and how they apply to deep diving. Just as with

Depth (Feet)	Pressure (Atmospheres) (Absolute)	Reduction of Air Supply	Navy No Decompression Limits (Minutes)	Ultrasound No Decompression Limits (Minutes)	Decompression Stops Needed On Single Tank	Safe Emergency Ascent Possibilities	Divers First Physically Notice Nitrogen Narcosis
30 (33)	2	1/2	None	205	Not Needed	Very Easy	None
60 (66)	3	1/3	60	50	Unlikely	Easy	Some Divers
100 (99)	4	1/4	25	20	Possible	Difficult	Many Divers
130 (132)	5	1/5	10	5	Very Possible	Very Difficult	Most Divers

Fig. 10-2 *Some of the variables to consider in deep diving.*

all diving experiences, you should prepare properly and completely, dive conservatively, and have an understanding of safety procedures. The material presented here is intended to help you to make informed decisions about deep diving (Fig. 10-2). Figure 10-2 details some of the variables to be considered as you dive deeper. As pressure in atmospheres and no-decompression limits do not correspond exactly, both depths are provided.

Deep Diving Conditions
AIR CONSUMPTION AND BREATHING RESISTANCE

Air leaving the scuba tank and going into a diver's lungs underwater must counteract the ambient pressure for the diver to breathe effortlessly. The deeper the dive, the denser the inhaled air must be per breath to neutralize the effects of increasing depth. Because more air molecules per breath are utilized to maintain this increased density, deeper dives shorten the duration of the air supply.

Many factors influence the rate of air consumption, making it difficult to precisely calculate. These factors include the diver's physical size, experience, fitness, and breathing habits, plus the physical and emotional stress of the dive. Swimming or work load, water temperature and depth, breathing resistance, and air losses due to leaks, and buoyancy control also affect available air supply. Figure 10-3 illustrates the average impact of depth on air consumption.

It is important to constantly monitor both the air supply and the bottom time of both members of the buddy pair and be observant of the bottom time cutoff point or a pre-agreed cutoff point based upon remaining available air. When the first member of the buddy team reaches the air cutoff point, the dive activities are terminated and the ascent is initiated. The air cutoff point needs to take into consideration such factors as depth, individual air consumption, decompression obligation and safety stops, plus surface swimming requirements. Depending upon surface conditions, it may be safer to return to the shore or the boat breathing from a regulator rather than utilizing the snorkel. However, in calm surface conditions, the diver may wish to conserve tank air and utilize the snorkel returning to the boat or

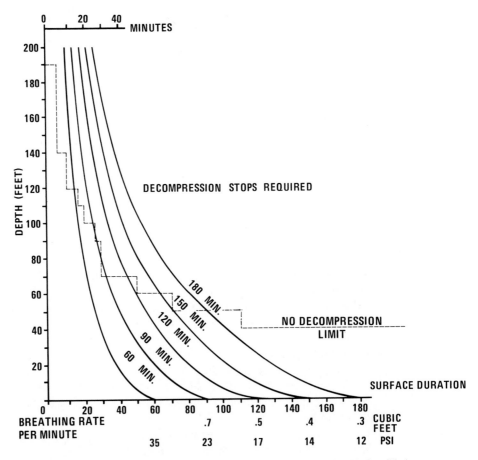

NOTE: This chart is based on a standard steel cylinder of 71.2 cubic feet filled to maximum pressure of 2475 psi and leaving 400 psi as a reserve.

Fig. 10-3 How air consumption varies depending on the depth of your dive.

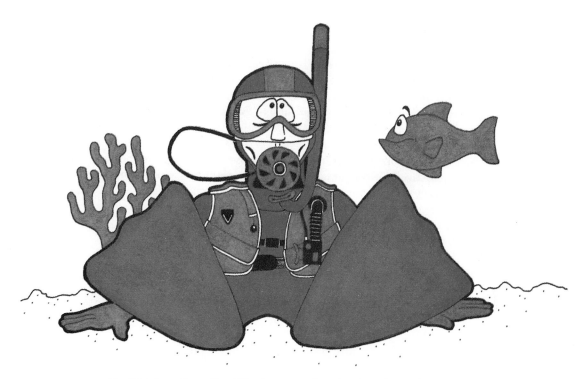

Fig. 10-4 *Sometimes it's difficult to get a breath when diving deeper if you are not using the appropriate equipment.*

beach. Different areas have differing philosophies regarding air conservation. Some would have the diver return to the boat with 500 psi remaining in the tank, while some instructors like to see their divers reach the safety stop with 500 psi remaining. The primary objective here is for the diver to reach an area of relative safety with a reasonable amount of air still remaining in the tank.

Breathing resistance, like air consumption, also increases with depth (Fig. 10-4). Greater depth and increasing pressures mean that the denser air must be moved through the regulator and the diver's airways. It is possible for divers to demand more air than some regulators can apparently supply under extreme conditions. These conditions include greater depths (generally over 100 feet), low tank pressures (less than 500 psi), rapid breathing rates, and poor regulator maintenance. Accident reports reveal that many so-called "out-of-air" situations actually occur when divers exceeded the performance capability of their regulators by diving under these conditions.

ENVIRONMENT

During deeper dives, surface conditions such as chop, surf, surge, or currents are normally not a factor with the exception of the entry/exit phase and safety decompression stops. Caution needs to be exercised when moving relative to the prevailing currents because the bottom and surface currents may run in different directions and at different speeds. It is advised that divers making deep dives do not cover a great deal of horizontal distance. Surfacing far from the starting point may require the expenditure of valuable energy needed to successfully return to the exit point and may actually increase the likelihood of decompression sickness.

Wet suits provide less warmth and buoyancy as depth increases because the increased pressure compresses the material. The loss of protection combined with colder water temperatures causes you to lose more heat, and therefore utilize more energy to produce body warmth. You may need to use a thicker wet suit and add hood, boots, and gloves when making a deep dive if these are not normal components of your diving attire. The increased depth also results in a loss of buoyancy, which will require adjustment of your buoyancy compensator (BC) when you reach depth.

Divers who routinely make deep dives in colder waters generally select a dry suit and appropriate undergarments. This is the correct choice because divers who are warm and comfortable handle the physical and emotional stresses better than those who are cold and bold. Air required for dry suit inflation is normally minimal for the experienced dry suit diver and not necessarily a consideration when selecting a suit for deep diving.

Sunlight, significantly filtered by greater depths, provides less available light and less apparent color. This depends upon a great many factors including the intensity of the sunlight (position of the sun or the time of day), actual depth, and clarity of the water. Turbid water combined with great depths may result in a tremendous reduction in ambient light at depth. These environmental conditions are shown in Fig. 10-5.

Even though the majority of aquatic life exists in the shallower waters, there are some fish, shells, corals, and other animals that live only at greater depths.

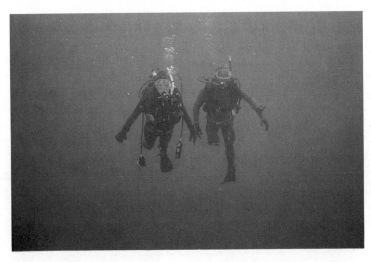

Fig. 10-5 *On the deep dive, the color and light intensity is diminished.*

DECOMPRESSION SICKNESS

Decompression sickness is a significant problem of deeper diving. Contrary to popular myth and misconception, all divers carry some decompression obligation regardless of depth or duration. On dives generally considered to be within the "no-decompression limits," the decompression obligation is met through a controlled ascent combined with a precautionary, "safety," stop of 3 to 5 minutes duration at a depth between 10 and 20 feet. Decompression and decompression sickness are dealt with in greater detail later in this chapter.

NITROGEN NARCOSIS

Nitrogen narcosis is a euphoric or lethargic condition brought on by breathing the high partial pressures of nitrogen in compressed air. The susceptibility and severity of this condition is increased by an increase in carbon dioxide. Also called "rapture of the deep," nitrogen narcosis creates situations that affect the deep diver to the extent that he or she may no longer be reliable or effective as a buddy. This condition, known as "behavioral toxicity," can severely compromise the safety of the diver and buddy. Although the exact mechanism is not completely understood, it is well documented that all deep divers are intellectually and physically impaired to varying degrees at depth. In some divers, the effects of nitrogen narcosis may be observed at depths of 60 feet, but most divers must approach 100 feet to be observably impaired, with the impairment significantly worsening with increased depth. Symptoms include loss of judgment and skill, false sense of well-being, lack of concern for safety, difficulty with time required to accomplish psychomotor tasks, and foolish behavior or inappropriate actions. The effects of nitrogen narcosis have been compared to those of alcohol intoxication—"Martini's Rule;" the two conditions are similar in that both degrade signal transmission along neural channels, both are dose-response related, and both have adaptive elements. Fig. 10-6 illustrates some of the progressive effects of nitrogen narcosis.

The effects are highly individual in nature and, in most cases, cannot be anticipated. The same diver may exhibit different signs from day to day and they may vary extensively from diver to diver. Narcosis will also be variable with environmental conditions. Extensive and recent diving experience and good physical condition tend to decrease some of the effects of nitrogen narcosis, while the use of drugs (including alcohol) and fatigue have definite adverse effects.

Divers exhibiting behavior inconsistent with safe diving should be considered to be suffering from the effects of nitrogen narcosis and brought to shallower water immediately. There are no apparent aftereffects. The effects of nitrogen narcosis are best avoided by diving to reasonable depths, being physically fit, using recently practiced and reinforced skills, using properly maintained equipment, and, above all, taking it slow and easy.

OTHER HAZARDS

Several other hazards that apply to all diving situations may be more significant for those who make deep dives. These include:

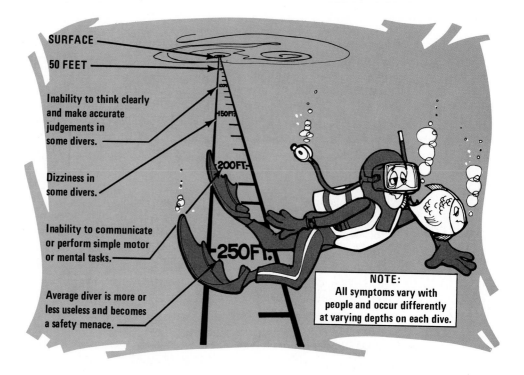

Fig. 10-6 *Nitrogen narcosis effects.*

1. Carbon dioxide excess
2. Drug use
3. Use of alcohol before diving
4. Cold and fatigue
5. Stress

In addition to being general hazards in diving, each of these can be a predisposing factor in decompression sickness (the bends), nitrogen narcosis, and other problems such as oxygen toxicity.

Deep Diving Preparation

Careful preparation will greatly improve the safety and enjoyment of the deep dive. Personal fitness, training, experience, planning, communications, and equipment all need to be superior and common practice for all dives, especially for those to deeper depths.

It is particularly important in deep diving to avoid harmful habits, including the use of any type of drugs, tobacco, and alcohol. No alcohol, in any form, should be consumed for at least 12 hours prior to a dive. If you regularly take some type of medication and are familiar with the potential side effects, its continued use should not be a particular problem provided you are careful and both you and your buddy are aware of the potential effects. Divers should never be under the influence of any substance that could potentially compromise the safety of the diver or buddy. If you have any doubts, consult a doctor familiar with hyperbaric medicine.

DIVE PLANNING

The dive plan is a tool you should use for safer and more enjoyable diving. A dive plan can be very simple and verbally handled between two buddies for most dives. But, when making dives with a greater degree of risk, such as deep diving, the dive plan needs to be more detailed, with some parts of it being written (Fig. 10-7).

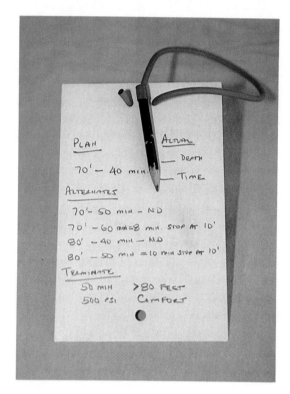

Fig. 10-7 *The dive plan recorded on the back of the dive slate, which should be a standard piece of equipment on a deep dive.*

Your first step is to find a buddy and decide on a time and place for the dive, along with a dive objective. You and your buddy should work out details of who, what, when, where, why, and how. Some aspects of the dive plan need particular attention for a deep dive:

1. Notify someone who is not going with you of your dive plans.
2. Select a simple objective for the dive.
3. Locate the nearest operational chamber and the quickest way to reach it. You should also know the number of the Divers Alert Network (DAN), which in the United States and Canada is 919-684-8111. This is an organiza-

tion that provides 24-hour telephone assistance for the treatment of diving accidents.

4. Carefully check weather and sea conditions.

5. Work out and record a decompression plan with an alternate plan in case you go over your time or depth.

6. Establish strict criteria for terminating the dive: Tank pressure (minimum); depth (maximum); time (maximum); and comfort.

7. Reserve the right to make the decision not to dive at any time, based on changing personal, medical, or environmental conditions.

COMMUNICATIONS

Communication methods are limited for recreational divers by either the cost or the ineffectiveness of most electronic and mechanical devices. You and your buddy should definitely carry a slate and a pencil. These need to be carefully secured so they will not be lost during the dive. Pertinent information, particularly decompression and alternate plans, should be recorded on the back of the slate before the dive. The other side of the slate can be used for underwater communication.

The standard hand signals should be reviewed as part of your comprehensive predive procedures (Fig. 10-8). Personal or regional hand signals or those not considered a part of every diver's manual vocabulary should be reviewed prior to the dive. Additional methods of underwater communication can be employed, such as talking into an inflated glove or using bone conductance. Talking into an inflated light-weight glove can be very effective. The sound is easily transmitted into the water, and most speech can be understood at short range. Talking by bone conductance is accomplished by placing the regulator second stage firmly against your buddy's head and speaking loudly and distinctly into the regulator. If the regulator is directly against the skull and not insulated by hair or suit material, a short conversation is possible. Whichever method is chosen, practice is required to speak clearly in these situations. This can be accomplished by practicing speech into your snorkel.

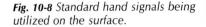
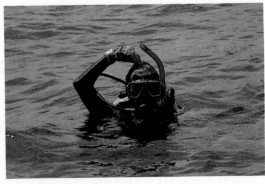

Fig. 10-8 Standard hand signals being utilized on the surface.

EQUIPMENT

Proper selection, use, and care of equipment is extremely important in deep diving. Changes to existing equipment and additional equipment may be required.

The scuba regulator should be single hose, top of the manufacturer's line, with a submersible pressure gauge. It should also have an alternate regulator or some other alternate source of air. You should carefully care for your regulator and take it to be professionally overhauled at least once a year. The alternate regulator is important for any out-of-air situation, but particularly when decompression is needed. No deep dive should ever be made without a submersible pressure gauge. It is the primary safety tool for planning and executing the safe deep dive.

Standard tanks, ranging in size from 70 or 80 cubic feet up to 100 cubic feet, are the most commonly used for sport diving, including deep diving.

Equipment that gives information becomes much more important on the deep dive (Fig. 10-9). In addition to the submersible pressure gauge, you and your buddy should have a depth gauge, watch, and compass. For added safety and efficiency, many divers use a bottom timer that automatically records the time of the dive. Serious deep divers use two depth gauges for each diver; a capillary gauge for accurate readings in shallow water during decompression, and a dial-reading depth gauge for easier reading at greater depths. Computers combine many of these functions and are becoming more widely used by many divers. However, as a precaution, the deep diver might consider carrying a complete console in addition to the computer so that all instrumentation is redundant.

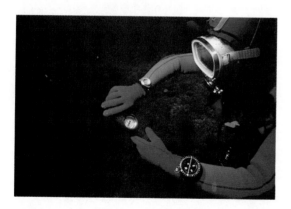

Fig. 10-9 *The properly equipped diver consults the console during the dive.*

Knowledge of your own dive limits and those of your equipment is extremely important when performing deep dives. Your level of experience should be the most important consideration in selecting the maximum depth and bottom time. You can plan and execute your dive using dive tables and a submersible pressure gauge or you can use a dive computer to provide more sophisticated information. In either case, you should be able to accurately calculate your dive time to remain within safe limits. During the dive, the equipment you use to monitor the necessary information should be accessible. It can become difficult to arrange and observe so many gauges and instruments, but you can conveniently place your instruments in a console that attaches to the submersible pressure gauge hose.

Other diving accessories should be kept at a minimum, consistent with the objective of the dive, so as not to get in the way and detract from a safe dive. The knife should be used as a safety tool. Also, due to the decreased light intensity, an underwater light, even in daytime, is often useful on a deep dive. You and your buddy should both carefully check over your own and the other's gear prior to any dive, as shown in Fig. 10-10. This buddy gear check should be done with particular care prior to a deep dive. All critical emergency skills and procedures should be reviewed and reinforced prior to initiating the dive.

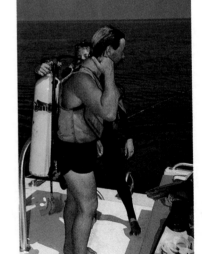

Fig. 10-10 Buddy gear check.

Surface Support Equipment

Under ideal conditions for deep diving, a surface support boat would be anchored above the dive site. This, of course, is not always possible, so much deep diving is done from shore. In using a boat in support of a deep dive, it should be anchored directly above the dive site, as shown in Fig. 10-11, with the anchor line used for descending and ascending. A decompression line separate from the anchor line, weighted, marked with dye or knots at 10-foot intervals, with an extra scuba unit with two second stages and extra weights, should also be hung over the side near the center of the boat. This will make decompression, if it is required, much safer and easier.

On board the boat, surface support personnel can handle equipment (e.g., additional air supplies and oxygen for emergencies) and act as safety divers. A dive-

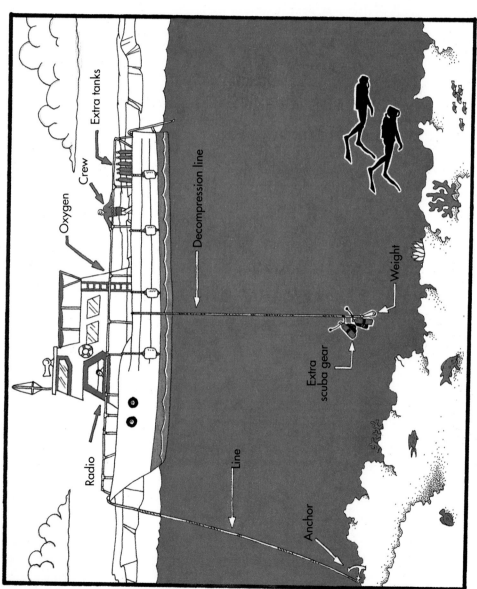

Fig. 10-11 *The diving boat set-up for the deep dive.*

master, qualified in deep diving, should supervise all aspects of the dive and have available a complete emergency plan including the location of the nearest operational recompression chamber.

The Deep Dive

After having set some reasonable depth limits based on your understanding of deep diving conditions and having made the necessary preparations for the deep dive, you are now ready to dive.

DESCENDING

At the surface do a final buddy check, making sure both you and your buddy are completely ready for the dive. You should equalize pressure in your ears at this time, even though you have not yet started your descent. When you are both ready you should go onto scuba and record the time on your slate. Next, completely deflate your BC and exhale to begin your descent.

If possible, descend all the way feet first, as shown in Fig. 10-12. The feet-first position makes it easier to equalize, provides better orientation, and allows for better descent control. If you have difficulty due to buoyancy, check your weight belt and air in your BC. If everything is in order you may want to pull yourself down the anchor line until compression offsets the buoyancy of the wet suit. If, however, the buoyancy is so great as to make the descent hard work, then resurface and adjust your weighting to neutral or slightly negative buoyancy at the surface. The problem with too much buoyancy is that you may have difficulty with too rapid an ascent at the end of the dive. In addition, any additional work or struggle connected with the descent will cause fatigue and CO_2 build-up, both of which compromise your safety.

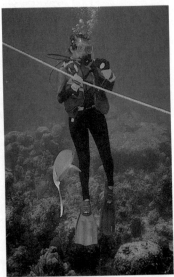

Fig. 10-12 *The feet-first descent is safest for the deep dive.*

If you are following the anchor line down, use it to help control your descent and to provide orientation. If either you or your buddy experience any difficulty, stop your descent until the problem is solved. Any recurring or significant problems may be cause to terminate the dive. If you are diving from shore, you can follow the bottom contour out into deep water. If sinking straight to depth in open water, proceed feet-first, taking it slow and easy, while using your bubbles and your buddy to help provide orientation. On all descents, use the BC to prevent yourself from becoming too negatively buoyant and continually clear your ears.

The rate of descent should be controlled by the slowest member of the buddy team. Ear clearing, comfort, and orientation should be the controlling factors. Never expect anyone to keep up with you—keep the buddy team together. Rapid descents can create severe problems with nitrogen narcosis. Be sure to maintain visual or physical contact with your buddy and use the anchor line, the bottom, or your bubbles to aid in orientation. As you descend, check your depth gauge to make sure you are not exceeding the depth of the planned dive.

AT DEPTH

When you arrive at the bottom, relax. Kneel or sit down and breathe easily while adjusting to the depth and becoming oriented. Check yourself, your gear, your instruments, your buddy, and the environment (Fig. 10-13). Communicate and make sure you are both comfortable and conditions are within the dive plan. Because of the depth, some sensations will change and you may notice a distinct difference in the sound of air coming from the regulator and your exhaust bubbles. Make sure that everything is under control before you and your buddy continue the dive. Any problems (equipment, narcosis, breathing rate, and so on) may require you to terminate the dive.

Inflate your BC for neutral buoyancy and be sure to maintain neutral buoyancy throughout the deep dive. Use a power inflator that enables you to use tank air to inflate your BC. This makes buoyancy adjustments quicker and easier to control.

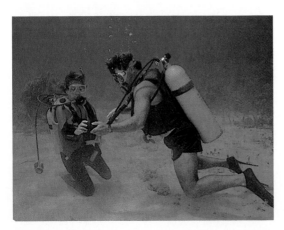

Fig. 10-13 *Checking over gear and conditions at depth.*

Maintain your contact and orientation with your buddy, with the line you use to descend, with the bottom, or by the use of your compass. Your pace should be slow and easy. The pace should be that of the slowest member of your buddy team. Always remain within effective reaction distance of your buddy. Your breathing should be slow, deep, and relaxed. Do not attempt any hard work at depth. If you feel yourself over-breathing, stop, breathe easy, think, and get control.

Note: It is particularly important to not make any dive plan changes that would increase depth or time while under the influence of nitrogen narcosis at depth.

Continue checking conditions, controlling buoyancy, and maintaining contact and orientation. Proceed with your dive objective, being prepared at any time to terminate the dive if any problem should develop or if you reach the limits of your plan. When you are ready to make a direct ascent to the surface, be sure you are neutrally buoyant and in contact with your buddy. Breathe easy, make a final check of instruments, record the time, and proceed to ascend.

ASCENDING

The ascent may be done on the anchor line, by following the bottom slope, or in open water, by using a combination of buoyancy control and swimming. It is also helpful to start the ascent by pushing off the bottom in open water, provided doing so will do no environmental damage.

Safe ascent rates are far slower than most divers realize. Most authorities now recommend an ascent rate of less than 60 feet per minute. The inflator or dump valve on your BC should be in your hand so you can vent off expanding air as you ascend (Fig. 10-14). By staying below your smallest bubbles and monitoring your

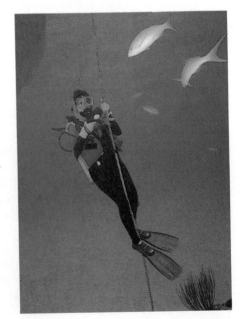

Fig. 10-14 *The proper, well-controlled ascent.*

gauges, you should be able to ascend at a rate not exceeding the recommended rate. Maintain contact with your buddy and keep your orientation by using the bottom, the anchor line, or your bubbles. The entire ascent should be very slow, easy, and controlled.

Your safety stop should be made at between 10 and 20 feet (most recommend 15 feet) for a period of 3 to 5 minutes. Though the anchor line or a special line hanging for safety stops may be present, you should be able to adjust your buoyancy so you can hang neutrally at your safety stop depth without using any devices.

As you approach the surface, continue to control your buoyancy and rate of ascent. If you are unable to maintain a controlled rate of ascent, use the anchor line or flare your body, as shown in Fig. 10-15. A controlled ascent rate fulfilling all decompression obligations is essential if deep diving is to be done safely and enjoyably.

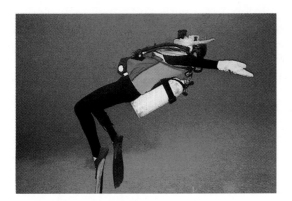

Fig. 10-15 *Flaring to slow ascent rate.*

Decompression

Although the actual mechanism of decompression sickness (DCS) is poorly understood, the fact that decompression obligations come with every scuba dive has been known for many years. The amount depends upon a variety of factors including the depth and duration of the dive. If the quantity of nitrogen dissolved in the tissues and blood exceeds a certain critical amount, divers must ascend slowly or make stops along the way to allow their tissues to remove the excess nitrogen. If this is not done, nitrogen bubbles will remain in the blood and tissues after the dive and cause DCS.

Recent research using Doppler ultrasound bubble detection equipment indicates that all decreases in pressure cause the formation of "silent bubbles" from nitrogen coming out of solution. The U.S. Navy Decompression Tables assume that the bubbles stay in solution as long as the partial pressure of nitrogen is not reduced by more than one-half and do not account for the silent bubbles. A careful and conservative approach while planning your dive decreases the likelihood of DCS (Fig. 10-16).

DECOMPRESSION SICKNESS

It is generally thought that DCS is the result of inadequate elimination of inert gas, principally nitrogen, from the diver's system. These gasses are usually removed from the diver's body when they come out of solution through the alveoli of the lungs and are harmlessly exhaled. If, however, conditions are such that the gasses are not eliminated from the body innocuously through the respiratory process, the gas may come out of solution in bodily tissues and result in DCS.

Causes of DCS may include exceeding the standard tables, deep dives following shallow dives, exceeding the acceptable rates of ascent, missing decompression stops where the dive profile dictates such stops, or multiday, multilevel diving where the diver's physiology simply cannot handle the excessive saturation of inert gasses over an extended period of time. For a number of cases of DCS, however, the cause of the disease is simply inexplicable and the disease simply is present.

Specific factors that may make an individual more susceptible to DCS include advanced age, obesity, fatigue, dehydration, alcohol or drug use, smoking, poor physical conditioning, illness, heavy work, cold diving, or impaired respiratory function from any chronic disease.

Symptoms

For many years it has been felt that one of the ways to differentiate between DCS and arterial gas embolism was the time that symptoms started. For example, if the injured diver started to show symptoms within 10 minutes of surfacing it was readily believed that the problem was arterial gas embolism. On the other hand, if

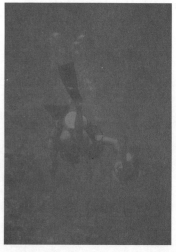

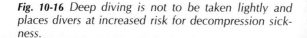

Fig. 10-16 *Deep diving is not to be taken lightly and places divers at increased risk for decompression sickness.*

symptoms did not start until the diver had been surfaced for 10 minutes or more, then it was thought it was safe to presume the problem was DCS. Based on the work of physicians in the United States and Great Britain we now know that a problem known as *patent foramen ovale* may accelerate the presence of symptoms of DCS and may also lead to the presence of symptoms that might be confused with arterial gas embolism. Patent foramen ovale is a fault in the wall between the two upper chambers of the heart (Fig. 10-17). Given the physical changes to which the body is exposed during diving, with this defect some of the inert gas bubbles in the circulation that might have been otherwise harmlessly eliminated from the bloodstream via the lungs may present a risk to the diver. Under certain circumstances and with the presence of this fault, the inert gas bubbles pass directly to the blood circulating throughout the body and never get sent to the lungs for elimination. Instead, these small and otherwise harmless bubbles get circulated to the brain and cause stroke-like injury, which is something of a blend between arterial gas embolism (bubbles blocking vessels) and DCS (the bubbles consist of inert gas rather than air).

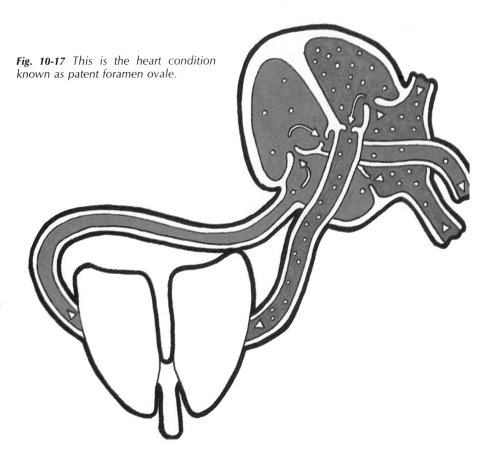

Fig. 10-17 *This is the heart condition known as patent foramen ovale.*

In general though, the symptoms of DCS start within a relatively short period of time following the last dive. Statistically, 63% of the divers with DCS show symptoms within 1 hour, and 89% within 6 hours. Only 7.5% of the DCS cases seen have onset delayed more than 6 hours but less than 24 hours. Since only 1% of DCS cases show signs or symptoms after 24 hours, it is generally felt that most situations that show symptoms after 24 hours following a dive are not DCS, unless flying after diving has been a factor (Fig. 10-18).

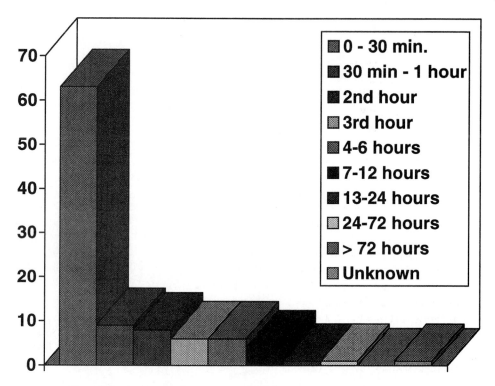

Fig. 10-18 *Time delay in signs and symptoms of DCS.*

Signs (what you observe) and symptoms (what the injured diver describes) of DCS are varied and are thought to be based on the location where the inert gas bubble formed in the body. The diver may be so severely injured as to be in cardiopulmonary arrest (though that typically happens with arterial gas embolism) or show as little as to simply be having "strange" feelings that cannot be accurately described. Any time that one has been diving and experiences any of the following, it would be wise to consult a physician knowledgeable in diving injuries or DAN:

- Pain
- Any change in level of consciousness
- Numbness, "pins and needles," tingling
- Vertigo or dizziness
- Visual disturbances

- Nausea/vomiting
- Hearing difficulty
- Speech difficulty
- Weakness
- Breathing difficulty
- Unusual swelling accompanied by any of the above
- A rash that cannot be accounted for from any other source

Though there is still much we do not understand about DCS, much of the pathophysiology of the disease is pretty well understood. Pathophysiology is a medical term that refers to the bodily changes that take place as a result of a particular disease. Nitrogen and to a lesser extent other inert gasses are the villains in DCS. When the gas comes out of solution, a number of events may take place. First, the very presence of bubbles may present a problem if they occur in too great a number. The offending bubbles may clog some of the very small vessels surrounding the alveoli of the lungs where gas exchange takes place and this may prevent gasses from being eliminated. If the bubbles occur in the structures or circulation of the spinal cord, the diver will experience various forms of nervous system signs and symptoms. If the bubbles lodge in the brain, signs and symptoms similar to a stroke may be present. The immune system of the body will attack these bubbles in much the same way any foreign substance is attacked and this process may cause blockage of the circulatory system and accompanying swelling. It may lead to a thickening of the blood. And, if sufficient segments of the circulatory system are blocked, the diver will actually be in a state of inadequate blood volume, which will simply accelerate and make more severe all of the other effects of the disease.

Treatment

First, the best treatment is prevention. Staying as fit as possible for diving is probably the first preventive step. Making sure that you are adequately rested and hydrated before you dive will be of significant help. Attempting to solve the hydration problem the morning of the dive is not the way to go. In order to help prevent DCS, all of the bodily tissues must be adequately hydrated. This process must begin not later than the night before the dive. Avoidance of substantial alcohol when diving will also slow down the dehydration process that often is a contributing factor to the development of DCS. Much has been written concerning flying after diving but when looking at the recreational scuba diver and susceptibility to DCS one also has to be concerned with flying before diving. Recognizing that most commercial airliners pressurize their cabins from 7000 to 9000 feet, the cardiorespiratory system has to work harder during a commercial flight. This includes an increased respiratory rate. When one understands that during the respiratory process water is exhaled along with CO_2, then we realize that commercial flights preceding diving activities contribute to the dehydration problem because water quantities beyond the norm are lost during the breathing process.

Limiting arduous work while diving as well as maintaining adequate body warmth will limit two of the known factors. Finally, whether you dive with computer or tables, a rigorous regard for the appropriate rules of whichever method is used will go a long way to help. "Safety Stops" following a dive, allow your body to release some of the remaining inert gas from the body at between 0.5 and 0.33 atmospheres gauge (1.5 to 1.33 ATA) and may be responsible for preventing far more cases of DCS than we will ever know. Finally, slowing down ascent rates will enable the body to more appropriately adjust to the gasses being eliminated, which might turn into bubbles if ascent was more rapid.

Without the presence of medically trained individuals, the only treatment that may be employed is keeping the diver in a position laying on the back (supine) (Fig. 10-19). It is imperative that 100% oxygen be administered beginning immediately after the injured diver is brought to the boat or to the beach. The most appropriate way to administer high concentrations of oxygen to the breathing diver is by the use of the oxygen powered, manually triggered demand valve unit, also simply referred to as the "demand valve." If a diver is not breathing, the same device may be used but should only be employed by those who have been trained in its use with non-breathing patients. For those not having this device available, mouth-to-mask ventilation should be employed and ideally should be supplemented by oxygen from a constant flow source (Fig. 10-20). The purpose of oxygen in DCS is twofold. First, by altering the partial pressure of oxygen in the injured diver, nitrogen may be eliminated from the system more effectively. Second, due to the problems associated with DCS as mentioned above, the oxygen "enriched" blood may limit or offset tissue damage that is likely to occur. If cardiopulmonary resuscitation is required (see Chapter 9), this must be initiated immediately and ventilations should be oxygen supplemented if possible. For the diver who is still breathing, the lower extremities may be slightly elevated in order to move more blood toward the most vulnerable organs.

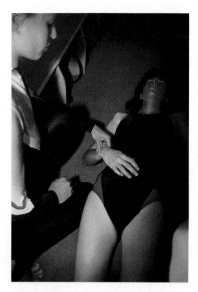

Fig. 10-19 *This is the position that the diver with suspected DCS should be placed in.*

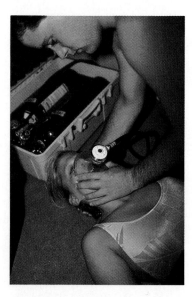

Fig. 10-20 *Diver being oxygenated with an oxygen-powered, manually triggered demand valve unit.*

If you are diving some distance from shore or assistance will be delayed in its arrival then the administration of fluids may be appropriate. If the injured diver is not in danger of choking, fluids can be given orally at a rate of about 8 oz every 15 minutes until the diver is delivered to a definitive care facility. If appropriately trained personnel are nearby, intravenous fluids should be administered. As soon as possible, the diver should be moved to the nearest facility with a recompression chamber for treatment. If you do not know where to take the patient you should either contact the local emergency medical services system or DAN (919-684-8111). Either of these sources will probably be able to direct you in delivering the injured diver to an appropriate medical facility. You should also attempt to learn as much as possible about the diver's profile—take notes! When transporting the diver to the medical facility, take the diver's gear and the "buddy" if possible. If the diving conditions were such that one diver is ill with DCS, there is a very good possibility that the buddy will be suffering from DCS as well—it may just take a bit longer.

The injured diver will be treated in a recompression chamber of either the monoplace or multiplace variety (Fig. 10-21). Though new types of chambers are being developed constantly, the principal benefit of the multiplace chamber is that an attendant can accompany the patient and administer care during the chamber dive. The typical treatments for DCS, depending upon the severity are Standard Treatment Table 5 or 6 (Figs. 10-22 and 10-23).

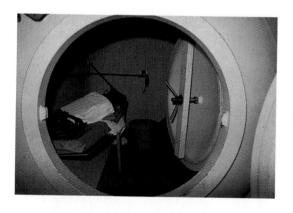

Fig. 10-21 *The multiplace chamber is the place where a patient can be cared for and taken to depth with someone medically trained in attendance.*

Prevention

A number of factors have been identified that appear to lead to increased risk of DCS. The more these risk factors or risk behaviors can be modified, the less likely it is that a diver will get decompression sickness. Among the risk factors/behaviors of significance are:

- Multiday, multilevel, repetitive dives
- Shallow dives preceding deep dives
- Deep dives—in excess of 100 feet
- Decompression dives

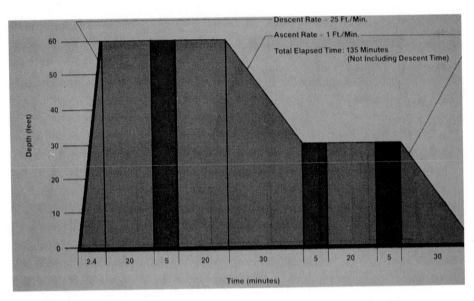

Fig. 10-22 *Table 5 is the table which at one time was used for "pain only" DCS symptoms. It is rarely used today except for subsequent treatments following the table below.*

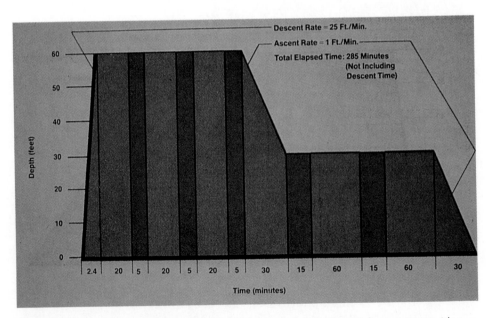

Fig. 10-23 *Table 6 is the initial table utilized in the treatment of DCS that presents with anything other than the most minor of symptoms.*

- Ascents in excess of 60 feet per minute
- Exceeding no-decompression limits for time or depth
- Dehydration
- Excessive alcohol consumption prior to diving
- Respiratory impairment
- Smoking
- Significant medical problems in the past
- Prior DCS
- Obesity
- Flying after diving

Regardless of what table or computer you are diving with, each dive actually is an experiment. All tables are based on one mathematical series of calculations or another. No tables have been established by physiologic evaluation of actual nitrogen in tissues. Instead, table theories are developed and the developers watch those diving with the tables to ascertain if they work in the manner the theorists projected they would.

No matter what table you choose, if any factor increases your chance of getting DCS, use the time limit specified for the next greater depth than the depth actually attained. Keep your ascent rate under 60 feet per minute. After every dive, stop at between 10 and 20 feet for between 3 and 5 minutes before surfacing.

Decompression Tables

A wide variety of decompression tables are in use worldwide as well as an even broader selection of dive computers. The editors have chosen to utilize the U.S. Navy Decompression Tables since these tables have withstood the test of time and are useful for teaching the basics of table utilization. We chose the Navy Tables in the Open Water text and use them here as well. There will always be controversy relative to the "safety" of one table over another but it must be recognized that all tables and computers have an inherent risk factor. When one exposes oneself to a decompression obligation, one is exposed to risk regardless of the table utilized. No table or instrument can guarantee absence of risk from decompression sickness. The U.S. Navy tables shown in Figs. 10-24 through 10-26 have certain definitions that need to be kept in mind. *Decompression* is a release from pressure and *decompression tables* are devised to allow for a controlled release from pressure to avoid the symptoms of DCS. To *recompress* is to put back under pressure. This is done during the treatment of DCS. *Chambers* are referred to as decompression, recompression, or hyperbaric chambers.

The bold black line and the numbers in parentheses on the no-decompression table in Fig. 10-24 provides recommended limits based on ultrasound studies. These limits are more conservative than the U.S. Navy Decompression Tables and provide an added margin of safety. The bold black line in the Residual Nitrogen Times table in Fig. 10-25 denotes U.S. Navy no-decompression limits. Any numbers to the left of the line are levels of nitrogen saturation that will require the use of the Standard Air Decompression Table to compute decompression times and depths (Fig. 10-26).

Depth (feet)	No-decompression limits (min)	Group Designation A	B	C	D	E	F	G	H	I	J	K	L	M	N	O
10		60	120	210	300											
15		35	70	110	160	225	350									
20		25	50	75	100	135	180	240	325							
25	(245)	20	35	55	75	100	125	160	195	245	315					
30	(205) NA	15	30	45	60	75	95	120	145	170	205	250	310			
35	(160) 310	5	15	25	40	50	60	80	100	120	140	160	190	220	270	310
40	(130) 200	5	15	25	30	40	50	70	80	100	110	130	150	170	200	
50	(70) 100		10	15	25	30	40	50	60	70	80	90	100			
60	(50) 60		10	15	20	25	30	40	50	55	60					
70	(40) 50			5	10	15	20	30	35	40	45	50				
80	(30) 40			5	10	15	20	25	30	35	40					
90	(25) 30			5	10	12	15	20	25	30						
100	(20) 25			5	7	10	15	20	22	25						
110	(15) 20				5	10	13	15	20							
120	(10) 15				5	10	12	15								
130	(5) 10				5	8	10									
140	10				5	7	10									
150	5				5											
160	5					5										
170	5					5										
180	5					5										
190	5					5										

Fig. 10-24 *No-decompression limits table.*

When using the decompression tables, *bottom time*, as shown in Fig. 10-27, is the time from leaving the surface until the diver starts a direct ascent back to the surface. *Depth* is figured as the deepest point reached during the dive. A repetitive dive is a second, or subsequent, dive made in less than 12 hours. Dives made more than 12 hours apart are counted as single dives. The time between repetitive dives is called the surface interval. Surface intervals are shown in the Residual Nitrogen Timetable (Fig. 10-26). As nitrogen is lost both during decompression and the surface interval, this time is taken into account when using the tables.

Residual nitrogen is that nitrogen left in your body after the dive. It could be compared to alcohol in the body that is gradually absorbed and consumed by the body until it is gone. In a similar manner, the residual nitrogen is gradually given off by your body until a normal nitrogen level is reached. To keep track of this residual nitrogen, after you have completed the first dive and a surface interval, the residual nitrogen is expressed as an amount of time you have already apparently spent at each possible depth before the next dive. This is provided in a table.

The decompression tables list *repetitive group letters*. These letters are arbitrary symbols established to help you compute how much nitrogen is still in your body. They start with "A," go through "O," then skip to "Z." Therefore, each letter of the alphabet utilized represents a certain amount of residual or leftover nitrogen you need to account for on repetitive dives.

The term *decompression schedule* is used by the Navy when referring to a particular depth and time in the decompression tables, such as, 130 feet for 15 minutes would be a 130/15 decompression schedule (Fig. 10-27). A *decompression stop* also is called *stage decompression*. These stops are set out in 10-foot increments in the decompression tables and are used to allow gradual nitrogen release. A *no-decompression dive* is one that does not require decompression stops according to the tables, even though decompression is going on during the ascent.

RESIDUAL NITROGEN TIMETABLE FOR REPETITIVE AIR DIVES

*Dives following surface intervals of more than 12 hours are not repetitive dives. Use actual bottom times in the Standard Air Decompression Tables to compute decompression for such dives.

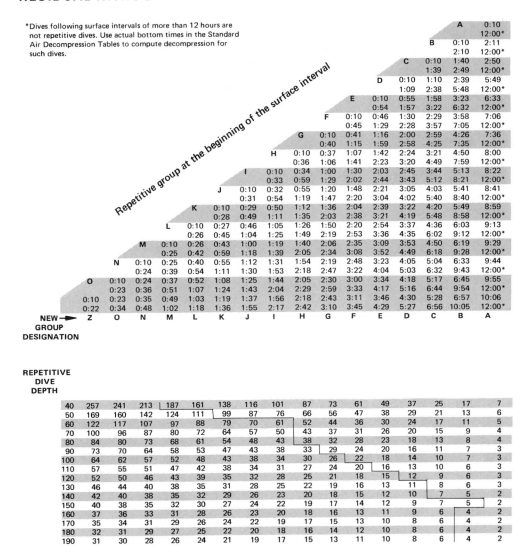

RESIDUAL NITROGEN TIMES (MINUTES)

Fig. 10-25 *Residual nitrogen timetable.*

U.S. NAVY STANDARD AIR DECOMPRESSION TABLE

Depth (feet)	Bottom time (min)	Time first stop (min:sec)	50	40	30	20	10	Total ascent (min:sec)	Repetitive group
40	200						0	0:40	*
	210	0:30					2	2:40	N
	230	0:30					7	7:40	N
	250	0:30					11	11:40	O
	270	0:30					15	15:40	O
	300	0:30					19	19:40	Z
	360	0:30					23	23:40	**
	480	0:30					41	41:40	**
	720	0:30					69	69:40	**
50	100						0	0:50	*
	110	0:40					3	3:50	L
	120	0:40					5	5:50	M
	140	0:40					10	10:50	M
	160	0:40					21	21:50	N
	180	0:40					29	29:50	O
	200	0:40					35	35:50	O
	220	0:40					40	40:50	Z
	240	0:40					47	47:50	Z
60	60						0	1:00	*
	70	0:50					2	3:00	K
	80	0:50					7	8:00	L
	100	0:50					14	15:00	M
	120	0:50					26	27:00	N
	140	0:50					39	40:00	O
	160	0:50					48	49:00	Z
	180	0:50					56	57:00	Z
	200	0:40				1	69	71:00	Z
	240	0:40				2	79	82:00	**
	360	0:40				20	119	140:00	**
	480	0:40				44	148	193:00	**
	720	0:40				78	187	266:00	**
70	50						0	1:10	*
	60	1:00					8	9:10	K
	70	1:00					14	15:10	L
	80	1:00					18	19:10	M
	90	1:00					23	24:10	N
	100	1:00					33	34:10	N
	110	0:50				2	41	44:10	O
	120	0:50				4	47	52:10	O
	130	0:50				6	52	59:10	O
	140	0:50				8	56	65:10	Z
	150	0:50				9	61	71:10	Z
	160	0:50				13	72	86:10	Z
	170	0:50				19	79	99:10	Z
80	40						0	1:20	*
	50	1:10					10	11:20	K
	60	1:10					17	18:20	L
	70	1:10					23	24:20	M
	80	1:00				2	31	34:20	N
	90	1:00				7	39	47:20	N
	100	1:00				11	46	58:20	O
	110	1:00				13	53	67:20	O
	120	1:00				17	56	74:20	Z
	130	1:00				19	63	83:20	Z
	140	1:00				26	69	96:20	Z
	150	1:00				32	77	110:20	Z
	180	1:00				35	85	121:20	**
	240	0:50			6	52	120	179:20	**
	360	0:50			29	90	160	280:20	**
	480	0:50			59	107	187	354:20	**
	720	0:40		17	108	142	187	455:20	**

Fig. 10-26 Standard air decompression table.

U.S. NAVY STANDARD AIR DECOMPRESSION TABLE

Depth (feet)	Bottom time (min)	Time to first stop (min:sec)	Decompression stops (feet)							Total ascent (min:sec)	Repetitive group
			70	60	50	40	30	20	10		
90	30								0	1:30	*
	40	1:20							7	8:30	J
	50	1:20							18	19:30	L
	60	1:20							25	26:30	M
	70	1:10						7	30	38:30	N
	80	1:10						13	40	54:30	N
	90	1:10						18	48	67:30	O
	100	1:10						21	54	76:30	Z
	110	1:10						24	61	86:30	Z
	120	1:10						32	68	101:30	Z
	130	1:00					5	36	74	116:30	Z
100	25								0	1:40	*
	30	1:30							3	4:40	I
	40	1:30							15	16:40	K
	50	1:20						2	24	27:40	L
	60	1:20						9	28	38:40	N
	70	1:20						17	39	57:40	O
	80	1:20						23	48	72:40	O
	90	1:10					3	23	57	84:40	Z
	100	1:10					7	23	66	97:40	Z
	110	1:10					10	34	72	117:40	Z
	120	1:10					12	41	78	132:40	Z
	180	1:00				1	29	53	118	202:40	**
	240	1:00				14	42	84	142	283:40	**
	360	0:50			2	42	73	111	187	416:40	**
	480	0:50			21	61	91	142	187	503:40	**
	720	0:50			55	106	122	142	187	613:40	**
110	20								0	1:50	*
	25	1:40							3	4:50	H
	30	1:40							7	8:50	J
	40	1:30						2	21	24:50	L
	50	1:30						8	26	35:50	M
	60	1:30						18	36	55:50	N
	70	1:20					1	23	48	73:50	O
	80	1:20					7	23	57	88:50	Z
	90	1:20					12	30	64	107:50	Z
	100	1:20					15	37	72	125:50	Z
120									0		
									2		
									6		
									14		
								5	25		
								15	31		
	60	1:30					2	22	45		
	70	1:30					9	23	55	89:00	O
	80	1:30					15	27	63	107:00	Z
	90	1:30					19	37	74	132:00	Z
	100	1:30					23	45	80	150:00	Z
	120	1:20				10	19	47	98	176:00	**
	180	1:10			5	27	37	76	137	284:00	**
	240	1:10			23	35	60	97	179	396:00	**
	360	1:00		18	45	64	93	142	187	551:00	**
	480	0:50	3	41	64	93	122	142	187	654:00	**
	720	0:50	32	74	100	114	122	142	187	773:00	**
130	10								0	2:10	*
	15	2:00							1	3:10	F
	20	2:00							4	6:10	H
	25	2:00							10	12:10	J
	30	1:50						3	18	23:10	M
	40	1:50						10	25	37:10	N
	50	1:40					3	21	37	63:10	O
	60	1:40					9	23	52	86:10	Z
	70	1:40					16	24	61	103:10	Z
	80	1:30				3	19	35	72	131:10	Z
	90	1:30				8	19	45	80	154:10	Z

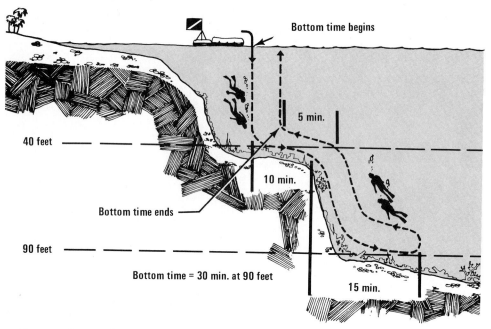

Bottom time begins

5 min.

10 min.

40 feet

Bottom time ends

90 feet

Bottom time = 30 min. at 90 feet

15 min.

Fig. 10-27 *Bottom time.*

USING THE TABLES

With the definitions in mind, some procedures should be reviewed. The maximum rate of ascent from compressed air scuba dives is 60 feet per minute; that is, 1 foot per second, which is a very slow rate. It can be gauged by staying behind the smallest bubbles and using your watch and depth gauge combination. This is the rate for the U.S. Navy, but your ascent rate would be better to be 20 to 40 feet per minute in water less than 60 feet. You can monitor that rate of ascent by utilizing your depth gauge and watch or many modern diving computers indicate your ascent rate.

When you use the decompression tables, *always round off both time and depth to the next greater time or depth*. Using the ultrasound limits will provide an added margin of safety. If you use the limits to the right of the bold line, there is no built in safety factor and it may put you in a potentially dangerous situation.

The no-decompression limits, shown in Fig. 10-28, should be used by recreational divers to avoid decompression. Even though a dive is a "no-decompression dive" there is still residual nitrogen in the diver's system. All dives to less than 33 feet are "no-decompression" dives. Even dives of 30 feet for over 205 minutes, however, require a decompression stop. Such a profile would be possible utilizing surface supplied air. Though not a recreational dive, the deepest a diver can go without a decompression stop is 190 feet with an allowable bottom time of 5 minutes. Since it would take nearly 5 minutes to reach 190 feet, there is little time to do anything once the depth is reached.

Depth (feet)	No-decompression limits (min)		A	B	C	D	E	F	G	H	I	J	K	L	M	N	O
																Group Designation	
10			60	120	210	300											
15			35	70	110	160	225	350									
20			25	50	75	100	135	180	240	325							
25	(245)		20	35	55	75	100	125	160	195	245	315					
30	(205)	NA	15	30	45	60	75	95	120	145	170	205	250	310			
35	(160)	310	5	15	25	40	50	60	80	100	120	140	160	190	220	270	310
40	(130)	200	5	15	25	30	40	50	70	80	100	110	130	150	170	200	
50	(70)	100		10	15	25	30	40	50	60	70	80	90	100			
60	(50)	60		10	15	20	25	30	40	50	55	60					
70	(40)	50		5	10	15	20	30	35	40	45	50					
80	(30)	40		5	10	15	20	25	30	35	40						
90	(25)	30		5	10	12	15	20	25	30							
100	(20)	25		5	7	10	15	20	22	25							
110	(15)	20			5	10	13	15	20								
120	(10)	15			5	10	12	15									
130	(5)	10			5	8	10										
140		10			5	7	10										
150		5			5												
160		5				5											
170		5				5											
180		5				5											
190		5				5											

Fig. 10-28 *No-decompression limits.*

All depths in the U.S. Navy Decompression Tables are in feet. All times in the decompression tables are in minutes with the exception of the surface interval table, which uses hours and minutes. Decompression stops are at 10-foot intervals. The deepest stop is at 50 feet and the shallowest is at 10 feet. When you are decompressing, the chest should be at the depth of the decompression stop.

The minimum surface interval used in the U.S. Navy Tables is 10 minutes. If dives are made less than 10 minutes apart, then the times of the two dives are added together and the greatest depth of the two dives is used to compute decompression.

An exception to the U.S. Navy Decompression Tables occurs when a repetitive dive is made to the same or greater depth than the previous dive, and the surface interval is short enough that the residual nitrogen time is greater than the actual bottom time of the previous dive. In this case, add the actual bottom time of the previous dive to the actual bottom time of the repetitive dive and decompress for the total bottom time and the deepest depth. For example, a dive was made to 70 feet for 50 minutes, with a surface interval of 30 minutes, and a repeat dive to 70 feet for 40 minutes is planned. The first dive left the diver in the "J" group. Following the repetitive dive table for a "J" group diver with a 30-minute surface interval to return to 70 feet, we find the residual nitrogen time is 57 minutes. Therefore, instead of adding the 57 minutes from the table, we use the actual bottom time for the first dive (50 minutes) and add it to the planned bottom time (40 minutes), for a total bottom time of 90 minutes at 70 feet. This puts the diver into a decompression situation requiring a decompression stop of 23 minutes at 10 feet. However, if the 57 minutes from the table were used, the diver would have to decompress for 33 minutes at 10 feet.

Depth (feet)	No-decompression limits (min)	A	B	C	D	E	F	G	H	I	J	K	L	M	N	O
								Group Designation								
10		60	120	210	300											
15		35	70	110	160	225	350									
20		25	50	75	100	135	180	240	325							
25	(245)	20	35	55	75	100	125	160	195	245	315					
30	(205) NA	15	30	45	60	75	95	120	145	170	205	250	310			
35	(160) 310	5	15	25	40	50	60	80	100	120	140	160	190	220	270	310
40	(130) 200	5	15	25	30	40	50	70	80	100	110	130	150	170	200	
50	(70) 100		10	15	25	30	40	50	60	70	80	90	100			
60	(50) 60		10	15	20	25	30	40	50	55	60					
70	(40) 50			5	10	15	20	30	35	40	45	50				
80	(30) 40			5	10	15	20	25	30	35	40					
90	(25) 30			5	10	12	15	20	25	30						
100	(20) 25			5	7	10	15	20	22	25						
110	(15) 20				5	10	13	15	20							
120	(10) 15				5	10	12	15								
130	(5) 10				5	8	10									
140	10				5	7	10									
150	5				5											
160	5					5										
170	5					5										
180	5					5										
190	5					5										

Fig. 10-29 *No-decompression limits based on ultrasound studies.*

This exception occurs because it is not possible to build into the U.S. Navy Decompression Tables every conceivable combination of dives. If you disregard this exception and handle the tables in the normal manner, rather than by the procedure listed here, your error will be on the safe side, as you will be decreasing your diving time if you are making no-decompression dives, or increasing the amount of time you spend decompressing.

AVOIDING DECOMPRESSION STOPS

There are several ways you can effectively use the decompression tables and deal with the problem of decompression. Making the first dive the deeper dive aids in decompression because each successive shallower dive will actually be helping you decompress. Also, the procedure of going to maximum depth first during any one dive, spending a limited time there, and then moving to shallow water, aids in decompression.

Diving to less than 33 feet usually does not require decompression stops, and repeated dives can be made in this depth range without significant concern about decompression. If deeper dives have been made earlier in the day, you should make subsequent dives in this lesser depth range. Making surface intervals between dives as long as possible also will aid in eliminating nitrogen and increase diving safety.

Recreational divers should not devise their own system for modifying the U.S. Navy Decompression Tables. The Navy has a proven system for what they call "cold or arduous" dives. This system can be used to modify the tables for any factor that might increase the likelihood of decompression sickness. The procedure is to use the next greater depth and time rather than that actually indicated by the dive.

This may cause you to decompress when you otherwise would not have done so, or it may decrease your dive time. It also provides that needed margin of safety. In addition, most divers today make the safety or precautionary stop previously discussed even when decompression stops are not required.

Recommended no-decompression limits that are based on ultrasound studies are illustrated in Fig. 10-29. The ultrasound limit for each depth is listed to the left of the bold line. These limits are also listed in parentheses in the "no-decompression limits (min)" column. Using the ultrasound limits provides an added margin of safety, since these limits are more conservative than the U.S. Navy's for each depth. For example, if the maximum depth of your first dive is 50 feet, the U.S. Navy's no-decompression limit is 100 minutes, and your repetitive group designation is "L." If you are a Navy diver between the ages of 18 and 25 and you are in excellent physical condition, this limit may be appropriate. Otherwise, you may be jeopardizing your safety by using this limit. If you dive to this depth for 70 minutes, as recommended by the ultrasound time limit, you will be well within a safe no-decompression time. Various ways of avoiding decompression dives are summarized in the box.

Ways to avoid decompression
_____

Make the first dive the deepest.
During each dive, go to maximum depth, spend limited time there, then move to shallower water.
Dive in water shallower than 33 feet.
Extend the surface interval time.
Use only proven dive tables.
Dive conservatively.

High-Altitude Diving

There are some special situations concerning deep and decompression diving that you should understand. The decompression tables were developed for diving in salt water at sea level. This is also true for nearly all other diving tables available to recreational divers. Therefore, they are not designed for fresh water lakes at high altitudes. As fresh water is slightly less dense than salt water, there will be a slight error on the safe side when you use the decompression tables in fresh water, if that fresh water is at, or near, sea level.

Several tables have been released for altitude diving. Most are simply mathematical computations modifying existing sea level tables. However, the Canadian DCIEM table D seems to offer some safe tables for use at altitudes above 999 feet. You should carefully review all standard and altitude tables before you dive in lakes at high altitudes and, at all times, use large safety margins.

Flying after Diving

There are few issues in recreational diving that have been more controversial than the hours that should elapse before one flies following the final dive. The consensus seems to put the burden of the decision largely on the diver based upon some suggestions for safety. To be as safe as possible, you should probably wait 24 hours after your last dive before you fly. In some cases, this guideline may be impractical. You should be aware, however, that flying within 12 hours of a no-decompression dive, and within 24 hours of a decompression dive, increases your risk of developing DCS. Most commercial airliners and private jets are not pressurized to sea level pressure. They maintain a cabin pressure of approximately 8000 feet, or about 10.9 psi. A loss of cabin pressure would probably cause the bends. As a general guideline you should wait at least 12 hours and, if at all possible, 24 hours before you fly. This conservative guideline may not totally eliminate your risk of developing the bends.

Bounce Dives

A "bounce dive" usually refers to a deep dive made very quickly. Such a dive might be made to check an anchor or pick up a piece of equipment. The bounce dive must be counted just as any other scuba dive as far as decompression requirements are concerned. Recreational divers also do a great deal of "multilevel" diving, as shown in Fig. 10-28. They may reach a maximum depth of 95 feet on the dive, but spend most of their time at 60 feet and actually be at 40 feet during part of the dive. The U.S. Navy Decompression Tables do not allow for this mode of diving as the entire dive is counted at the greatest depth. Most dive computers account for this type of dive profile (see Chapter 1).

Decompression Procedures

The ideal method for decompressing from a deep dive is to use a decompression line hung from a boat or to use the boat's anchor line. If the boat rolls or pitches while you hang on the line, you must adjust your position so your chest never rises above the prescribed decompression stop depth. This potential risk points to the need to be able to maintain neutral buoyancy at a specific depth, as mentioned before. Alternatively, you can take a gentle swim at your decompression depth or, if possible, swim to an area of shallower water at your decompression depth and explore the bottom. A third method is to tie a light line to something on the bottom or anchor the line with a weight. The length of the line should be such that a float at the end of the line is at the decompression depth, as shown in Fig. 10-30. Setting your decompression line in this manner pretty well eliminates the problems connected with surface conditions.

Omitted decompression is when a diver is forced to skip or cut short a scheduled decompression stop. If you should omit a stop, for whatever reason, there is a prescribed procedure you are to follow. If there are no signs or symptoms of DCS and there is no recompression chamber available, you should lie down, breathe O_2 and drink fluids, such as water, while monitoring yourself for signs of DCS.

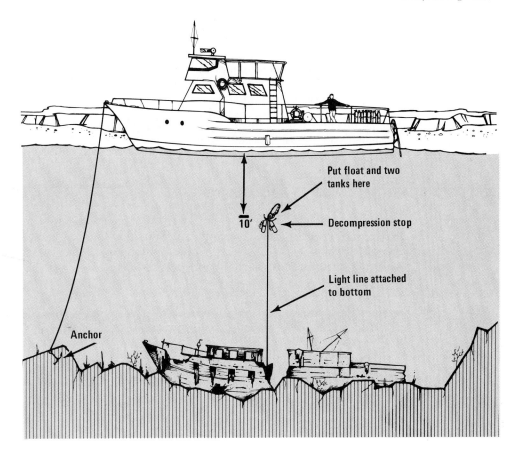

Put float and two tanks here

Decompression stop

Light line attached to bottom

10'

Anchor

Fig. 10-30 *Another approach to decompression and decompression stops is to rig your extra equipment and line from the bottom.*

Dive Planning with Decompression Tables

The tremendous importance of dive planning, particularly on a deep dive, has already been described and cannot be overemphasized. A crucial part of dive planning during the deep dive is to deal with decompression. The decompression tables can be used in a variety of ways to plan a dive and avoid or take the required decompression.

These dive planning methods include using the decompression tables in several ways:

1. To avoid decompression stops.
2. To stay within a particular decompression schedule or repetitive group.
3. To attain maximum depth or time on a limited air supply.
4. To make minimum decompression stops.

5. To make a particular dive and take whatever decompression stops are required.
6. To calculate the maximum time available on a second dive without decompression.
7. To calculate the minimum surface interval to avoid decompression.

Though this material has been based thus far on the U.S. Navy tables, the Appendix contains additional information on other tables that may be utilized, all of which are more conservative than the U.S. Navy tables.

Decompression Worksheets and Diagrams

Many different types of worksheets to record decompression requirements have been devised. Many are far too complicated to be useful in diving. A simple worksheet is shown in Fig. 10-31. This information can be listed either across the top or down the side of a 3″ × 5″ card or recorded in your dive log at the end of a day's diving.

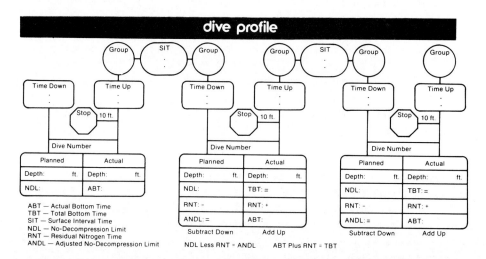

Fig. 10-31 *Dive Profile worksheet.*

Diagramming a dive is a useful tool to visualize the day's repetitive dives. These diagrams are most often used during training to make it clear how the procedures and calculations are handled. Two such diagrams are shown in Fig. 10-32.

Mixed Gas Diving

Very few issues in modern recreational scuba diving have led to more controversy than the possible use of mixed gases by recreational divers. Oxygen-enriched breathing mixtures have been used in the commercial, military, and scientific communities for many years but the great concern by many in the recreational scuba

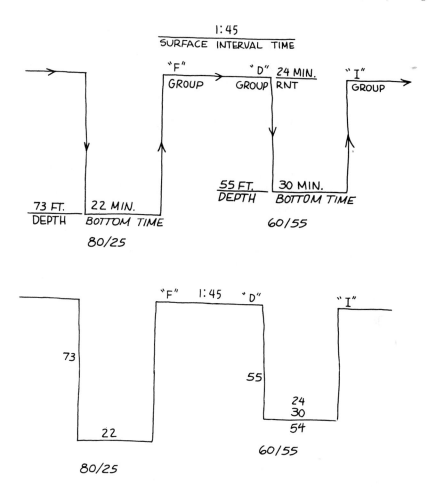

Fig. 10-32 *Dive diagrams.*

diving industry stresses that these diving environments usually impose rigid controls on divers utilizing mixed gases.

Much debate has taken place among the editors and reviewers of this book relative to the inclusion of this material in a recreational diving publication. However, our ultimate decision to include this material was based on the conclusion that to do otherwise would be like sticking our heads in the sand. Furthermore, at the time this book was in its final stages of development, one of the major U.S. diving agencies was recognizing oxygen-enriched diving as a high-risk specialty in much the same manner that cave and ice diving are recognized.

The editor would like to offer several precautions to the recreational diver considering mixed gas diving. First, do not ever undertake this type of diving without having undergone specialized training in the utilization of mixed gases. Diving with mixed gases possesses its own set of rules and tables with which the diver must be fully familiar before undertaking the sport. For the enriched gases that will be utilized by recreational divers, depth limitations are more conservative and no recreational diver utilizing mixed gasses should ever descend to a depth equal to or greater than 100 feet. A major concern has to do with the source of breathing gases. Under no circumstances should recreational divers attempt to prepare their own enriched diving gas mixtures. Cases where this has happened have led to the diver's death. Instead, after receiving complete training in mixed gas diving and familiarization with the necessity of proper gas mixing, secure your enriched breathing gases only from recognized sources of mixed gases for diving. Finally, consult the manufacturer of your scuba equipment to determine if the equipment is suitable for mixed gas diving. Some manufacturers will not warrant nor do they recommend that their equipment be utilized in the mixed gas diving environment.

MIXED GAS DIVING THEORY

The term *mixed gas,* refers to *any* breathing medium other than air. The mixed gas of choice may consist of nitrogen and oxygen in proportions other than those found in atmospheric air (whether it is produced by mixing individual gases or enriching atmospheric air with oxygen), or it may be a mixture of any of a variety of inert gases (i.e., helium, hydrogen, and so on) blended with oxygen. A mixed gas dive requires comprehensive preparation; complete planning and precise execution borne of understanding of the advanced concepts of mixed gas theory. There is little room in the use of any mixed gases for a cavalier attitude towards safety.

Nitrogen-Oxygen Mixtures

Nitrogen-oxygen mixtures are normally limited to relatively shallow depths (< 100 fsw). Air, the most commonly available mixture, can be used at these depths with relative safety and reliability with the appropriate level of knowledge, training, and preparation. Nitrogen narcosis is considered the major limiting factor for the use of air for deep dives (> 100 fsw). The depth (or pressure) at which narcosis symptoms first appear varies widely among individual divers and may vary from day to day or even dive to dive with the same person. The first observable signs and symptoms normally occur at a depth of 100 fsw. Experimental evidence, however, has shown that certain susceptible individuals exhibit significant neurologic deficits even at depths as comparatively low as 60 feet. These symptoms involve significant decrements in conceptual reasoning, reaction time, and dexterity increasing markedly with depth. The effects are likely to compromise the safety of the individual diver and other members of the dive group. Narcosis may affect the diver's behavior to the extent that he or she is no longer reliable nor effective as a buddy. The condition, known as *behavioral toxicity,* may be accentuated by a buildup of CO_2 from physical exertion, anxiety, or the influence of residual alcohol or other drugs.

The common term used for gas mixtures with a greater fraction of oxygen than air is *nitrox* or *enriched air nitrox (EANx).* The term is sometimes also confused with *nitrous oxide* or *"laughing gas."* Nitrous oxide has a completely different chemical formula (N_2O as compared with N_2O_2) and, because of its anesthetic properties, is obviously not compatible with safe diving. The term *safe air* has been recently applied to EANx. It has, in fact, been stated that EANx is not a mixed gas at all, but rather simply a safer form of atmospheric air. These statements are very misleading and, in actuality, incorrect. Nitrox *is*, indeed, a mixed gas requiring a level of preparation and understanding to a degree far beyond that required of air.

The N.O.A.A. Diving Program commonly uses a standard mixture of 32% oxygen and 68% nitrogen known as N.O.A.A. Nitrox I (NNI). A second standard mixture, known as N.O.A.A. Nitrox II (NNII), has been proposed having 37.5% oxygen and 62.5% nitrogen. There is currently some discussion as to the true applicability of the proposed NNII proportions and other mixtures are currently under consideration (i.e., 36% oxygen and 64% nitrogen). Depending on the mixing capabilities of the compressed gas source, any number of conceivable mixtures can be produced to give the desired extended bottom time or reduced decompression obligation. These mixes are commonly known as *optimal mixes*.

A nitrogen-oxygen mixture containing a higher fraction of oxygen than air (e.g., 32% oxygen/68% nitrogen) and, therefore, a lower proportion of nitrogen, may have a number of distinct advantages over air: (1) greater bottom times within the "no-stop" or "no-decompression" limits (Fig. 10-25); (2) reduced decompression obligations; (3) a *proportional* reduction in narcosis; and (4) a greater margin of reliability when used as air for multidive/multiday diving.

The problems associated with using an enriched air mix come from the increased oxygen fraction and the potentially toxic effects of high partial pressure oxygen. Due to potential for central nervous system (CNS) toxicity, it is suggested that safety-conscious divers limit the use of any EANx mix to no greater than 100 fsw. Carbon dioxide would, as previously discussed, reduce the diver's tolerance for oxygen toxicity and, therefore, predispose a working diver to potential O_2 seizures. Divers are advised to *always* choose the most conservative approach where safety is concerned.

Helium-Oxygen Mixtures

For diving to depths where the narcotic properties of nitrogen would seriously affect the performance and, potentially, compromise the safety of the diver, a mixture of helium and oxygen is generally preferred. The substitution of helium for nitrogen virtually eliminates the deleterious effects of narcosis at known diving depths. Helium, although virtually nonnarcotic, does, however, create its own set of problems.

In situations where working divers must use voice communications, helium creates a form of vocal distortion known as the *Donald Duck effect*, worsening progressively with increasing depth and gas density. Although marginally neutralized with experience, effective and intelligible speech can only be gained with the aid of a rather expensive electronic "unscrambler." Because of the significantly greater thermal conductivity of helium (six times that of air), heat loss is generally considered to be a problem especially in situations where the diver is surrounded by a helium atmosphere (i.e., saturation diving). The suspected potential for respiratory heat loss while breathing helium has been an area of significant concern and controversy for diving physiologists. Respiratory heat loss may, however, not be as significant as originally suspected, especially during the relatively short excursions while scuba diving.

Miscellaneous Gas Mixtures

Another alternative to nitrogen-oxygen and helium-oxygen blends is known as *tri-mix*. Tri-mix, a specific blend of helium, nitrogen, and oxygen, gives the diver the operational advantages of all three gases. It is superior over HeO_2 in reducing any significant respiratory heat loss while maintaining vocal integrity. It is preferred over nitrox blends in allowing the diver to retain some level of functional intellectual capability (due to the reduced nitrogen) during deep diving excursions.

Through the years, other more exotic gas mixtures and specific blends have been suggested and tried with varying degrees of success and failure. The use of other inert gases imposes severe limitations on reliability and safety.

GAS MIXING AND ANALYSIS

Errors in gas mixing can have serious ramifications and ultimately compromise the safety of the diver and buddy. It is always advisable to secure gas premixed from a reliable source. Never accept any gas mixture (even air) whose origin and exact content are suspect.

The oxygen content of all gas mixtures (other than air) must be analyzed by the diver prior to being used. Since most analyzers have the same frailties and are subjected to the same abuse as other forms of diving-related instrumentation, it would be wise and prudent to have a back-up. They are relatively expensive (in the range of $300 to $1,000). Each cylinder must be identified as to the specific analyzed mix and that should be entered into diver's log. This information should also be added to the diver's emergency assistance plan so that if treatment is necessary, the medical emergency facility can make decisions based upon recent exposures to elevated partial pressures of oxygen.

PLANNING

Mixed gas requires a much greater emphasis upon the concepts of risk management than air. For example, in order to avoid confusion with air, mixed gas cylinders should be dedicated and marked as to their exact contents. Various color schemes have been suggested and used. NOAA recommends that all nitrox cylinders have a 4″ oxygen-green band at the shoulders and be identified as "nitrox". The individual divers and surface support must be satisfied that all areas that may compromise the safety of the diver are identified and neutralized prior to the beginning of any diving activity. The old adage, "when in doubt . . . stay out" should certainly apply to mixed gas diving. This is no area for those bold divers with a cavalier attitude toward safety. You must choose and use all mixed gases wisely with wisdom borne of knowledge and practice.

Appendix

WATER TEMPERATURE PROTECTION CHART

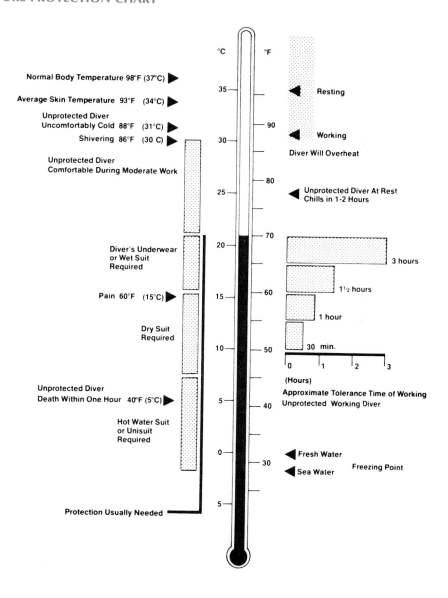

Normal Body Temperature 98°F (37°C) ▶

Average Skin Temperature 93°F (34°C) ▶

Unprotected Diver
Uncomfortably Cold 88°F (31°C) ▶

Shivering 86°F (30 C) ▶

Unprotected Diver
Comfortable During Moderate Work

Diver's Underwear
or Wet Suit
Required

Pain 60°F (15°C) ▶

Dry Suit
Required

Unprotected Diver
Death Within One Hour 40°F (5°C) ▶

Hot Water Suit
or Unisuit
Required

Protection Usually Needed

°C   °F

35 ——

90 ——

30 ——

80 ——

25 ——

70 ——

20 ——

60 ——

15 ——

50 ——

10 ——

5 ——

40 ——

0 ——

30 ——

5 ——

Resting ◀

Working ◀

Diver Will Overheat

Unprotected Diver At Rest ◀
Chills in 1-2 Hours

3 hours

1½ hours

1 hour

30 min.

0   1   2   3

(Hours)

Approximate Tolerance Time of Working
Unprotected Working Diver

Fresh Water ◀

Sea Water ◀   Freezing Point

263

Air Purity Standards

The U.S. Navy Diving Manual provides that air used in scuba operations must meet minimum standards of purity as established by the Commander Naval Medical Command. The standards applied by the U.S. Navy are as follows:

Oxygen concentration	20% to 22% by volume
Carbon dioxide	1,000 ppm maximum
Carbon monoxide	20 ppm maximum
Total hydrocarbons other than methane	25 ppm maximum
Particulates and oil mist	5 mg/m³ maximum
Odor and taste	Not objectionable

These standards are recognized as acceptable purity levels throughout the United States.

Archimedes Principle and Gas Laws

Archimedes Principle: Any object wholly or partially immersed in a liquid is buoyed up by a force equal to the weight of the liquid displaced. (A) A negatively buoyant body sinks in a fluid because the weight of the fluid it displaces is less than the weight of the body. (B) A neutrally buoyant submerged body remains in equilibrium, neither rising nor sinking, because the weight of the fluid it displaces is exactly equal to its own weight. (C) A positively buoyant submerged body weighs less than the volume of liquid it displaces. It will rise and float with part of its volume above the surface. A floating body displaces its own weight of a liquid.

Boyle's Law: If the temperature is kept constant, the volume of a gas will vary inversely as the ABSOLUTE pressure while the density will vary directly as the pressure. Since the pressure and volume of a gas are inversely related—the higher the pressure, the smaller the volume, and vice-versa. The formula for Boyle's Law is:

$$PV = C$$
$$\text{Where } P = \text{absolute pressure}$$
$$V = \text{volume}$$
$$C = \text{a constant}$$

Charles' Law: If the pressure is kept constant, the volume of a gas will vary directly as the ABSOLUTE temperature. The amount of change in either volume or pressure is directly related to the change in absolute temperature. For example, if absolute temperature is doubled, then either the volume or the pressure also is doubled. The formula for Charles' Law is:

$$PV = RT \text{ or } \frac{PV = R}{T}$$
$$\text{Where } P = \text{absolute pressure}$$
$$V = \text{volume}$$
$$T = \text{absolute temperature}$$
$$R = \text{a universal constant for all gases}$$

General Gas Law: Boyle's Law illustrates pressure/volume relationships, and Charles' Law basically describes the effect of temperature changes on pressure and/or volume. The General Gas Law is a combination of these two laws. It is used to predict the behavior of a given quantity of gas when changes may be expected in any or all of the variables. The formula for the General Gas Law is:

$$\frac{P_1 V_1}{T_1} = \frac{P_2 V_2}{T_2}$$

Where P_1 = initial pressure (absolute)
V_1 = initial volume
T_1 = initial temperature (absolute)
P_2 = final pressure (absolute)
V_2 = final volume
T_2 = final temperature (absolute)

Dalton's Law: The total pressure exerted by a mixture of gases is equal to the sum of the pressures of each of the different gases making up the mixture—each gas acting as if it alone was present and occupied the total volume. The whole is equal to the sum of its parts and each part is not affected by any of the other parts. The pressure of any gas in the mixture is proportional to the number of molecules of that gas in the total volume. The pressure of each gas is called its partial pressure (pp), meaning its part of the whole. Dalton's Law is sometimes referred to as "the law of partial pressures." The formula for Dalton's Law is:

$$P_{Total} = PPA + PP_B + PP_C. \ldots$$
and
$$PP_A = P_{Total} \times \frac{\% \, Vol._A}{100\%}$$

Where P_{Total} = Total absolute pressure of gas mixture
PP_A = Partial pressure of gas A
PP_B = Partial pressure of gas B
PP_C = Partial pressure of gas C

Henry's Law: The amount of a gas that will dissolve in a liquid at a given temperature is almost directly proportional to the partial pressure of that gas. If one unit of gas dissolves in a liquid at one atmosphere, then two units will dissolve at two atmospheres, three units at three atmospheres, etc.

Air Consumption Formula/Table (See p. 268)

Knowing your air consumption rate is very important. By determining your consumption rate at the surface, it becomes a simple matter to calculate what it will be at any given depth. Since pressure gauges are calibrated in pounds per square inch (psi), your consumption rate must be psi too. The formula is as follows:

$$\frac{PSI \div TIME}{33/33 + DEPTH/33}$$

PSI = psi consumed in timed swim at a constant depth.
TIME = Duration of timed swim.
DEPTH = Depth of timed swim.

EXAMPLE: A diver swims at a depth of 10 feet for 10 minutes and consumes 300 psi of air. You want to determine his surface consumption expressed in psi.

$$\frac{300 \text{ (PSI used)} \div 10 \text{ (Time)} = 30}{33/33 + 10 \text{ (Depth)}/33 = 43/33} = \frac{30 \times 33}{43} = \frac{990}{43} = 23.02$$

23.02 PSI = PSI CONSUMED PER MINUTE AT SURFACE

NOTE: Consumption rate must be recalculated if tank size is changed. See Table on p. 268.

Sport Diver Open Water U.S. Navy Dive Tables (See illustration on p. 269)

Comparison of Several Popular Dive Tables

Today, there are many dive tables available to the sport diver, derived from various theories and methodologies to determine the effect of saturated nitrogen, and all having the primary intent of ensuring safety of the sport diver.

The new sport diver will learn from the dive table advocated by the agency providing the diving instruction.

Below is a synopsis of the no-decompression limits for air dives at various depths taken from 40 to 100 feet so that the reader can see the differences and similarities among the tables.

Maximum No-Decompression Limit

Depth	(1) U.S. Navy	(2) DCIEM	(3) PADI RDP	(4) PADI Wheel	(5) NAUI Table	(6) NAUI DTC 2
40	200	175	140	140	130	130
50	100	75	80	80	80	80
60	60	50	55	55	55	55
70	50	35	40	40	45	45
80	40	25	30	30	35	35
90	30	20	25	25	25	25
100	25	15	20	20	22	22

To clarify the sources of these figures, the following is provided as a reference to the above and relates to the numbers appearing above the respective column:

1. U.S. Navy Air Decompression Table—Revision, May 1989.
2. Sport Diving Tables—Department of National Defence (Canada) and produced under license by Universal Dive Tectronics, Inc., 2340 Vauxhall Place, Richmond, BC, Canada V6V 1YB—1987.
3. Recreational Dive Planner—Diving Science & Technology Corp. and distributed by International PADI, Inc.
4. The Wheel—Diving Science & Technology (DSAT) and distributed by International PADI, Inc., 1985, 1986, 1987, and 1988.
5. Dive Tables—National Association of Underwater Instructors, 1990.
6. Dive Time Calculator II—National Association of Underwater Instructors, 1989.

To take this analysis further, we will assume that a dive team makes a dive to 60 feet for 40 minutes. The divers then return to the surface and have a surface interval time (SIT) of 3 hours, 20 minutes, following which the divers perform a second dive to 40 feet for 60 minutes. We compare how the divers are treated by each of the above tables relative to Repetitive Dive Group after dive No. 1, Residual Nitrogen Times if applicable, Dive Group at the beginning of the second dive, Maximum allowable bottom time on the second dive, and Repetitive Dive Group after dive No. 2.

Repetitive Dive Group* at the end of dive 1

	U.S. Navy	DCIEM	PADI RDP	PADI Wheel	NAUI Table	NAUI DTC 2
60 feet for 40 min	G	E	Q	Q	G	G

Residual Nitrogen at beginning of dive 2 after SIT

Depth	U.S. Navy	DCIEM	PADI RDP	PADI Wheel	NAUI Table	NAUI DTC 2
40 feet	25	40†	9	‡	25	25

Group Designation at beginning of dive 2

	U.S. Navy	DCIEM	PADI RDP	PADI Wheel	NAUI Table	NAUI DTC 2
3:20 SIT	B	N/A	A	A	C	C

Though the dive plan calls for a second dive for 60 minutes, the maximum adjusted no-decompression limit for the second dive is as follows:

Depth	U.S. Navy	DCIEM	PADI RDP	PADI Wheel	NAUI Table	NAUI DTC 2
40 feet	175	135	131	131	105	105

Group Designation at the end of dive 2

Depth	U.S. Navy	DCIEM	PADI RDP	PADI Wheel	NAUI Table	NAUI DTC 2
40 feet for 60 min	I	N/A	P	P	I	I

NOTE: Group designations is indicated N/A under the DCIEM table due to the unique way that repetitive dives are computed using their table.

*The Wheel and Recreational Dive Planner use the term pressure group (PG) rather than repetitive dive group and cannot be used to enter any table using the repetitive dive group designation, as the groupings are based on the research and theories of DSAT only. Users of the Wheel and the Recreational Dive Planner may use either interchangeably, as they are based on the same research and theories.
†Due to the methodology used by the DCIEM tables, this is an interpolated value.
‡The Wheel does not give residual nitrogen times.

Locating Your Nearest Recompression Chamber

The following numbers may be called 24 hours a day, 7 days a week. Physicians are on call and consultation can be provided on air embolism or decompression sickness cases. Each maintains a world-wide listing of recompression chambers.

Divers Alert Network
DAN
919-684-8111

U.S. Navy Experimental Diving Unit
EDU Duty Phone
904-234-4553

AIR CONSUMPTION TABLE AT DEPTH

DEPTH IN FEET

Surface	10	15	20	25	30	40	50	60	70	80	90	100	120	140	160
15	19.5	21.8	24.0	27.0	28.5	33.0	37.5	42.0	46.5	51	55.5	60	69	78	87
16	20.8	23.2	25.6	28.8	30.4	35.2	40.0	44.8	49.6	54.4	59.2	64	73.6	83.2	92.8
17	22.1	24.7	27.2	30.6	32.3	37.4	42.5	47.6	52.7	57.8	62.9	68	78.2	88.4	98.6
18	23.4	26.1	28.8	32.4	34.2	39.6	45.0	50.4	55.8	61.2	66.6	72	82.8	93.6	104.4
19	24.7	27.6	30.4	34.2	36.1	41.8	47.5	53.2	58.9	64.6	70.3	76	87.4	98.8	110.2
20	26.	29.0	32.0	36.0	38.0	44.0	50.0	56.0	62.0	68.0	74.0	80	92	104	116
21	27.3	30.5	33.6	37.8	39.9	46.2	52.5	58.8	65.1	71.4	77.7	84	96.6	109.2	121.8
22	28.6	31.9	35.2	39.6	41.8	48.4	55.0	61.6	68.2	74.8	81.4	88	101.2	114.4	127.6
23	29.9	33.4	36.8	41.4	43.7	50.6	57.5	64.4	71.3	78.2	85.1	92	105.8	119.6	133.4
24	31.2	34.8	38.4	43.2	45.6	52.8	60.	67.2	74.4	81.6	88.8	96	110.4	124.8	139.2
25	32.5	36.3	40.0	45.0	47.5	55.0	62.5	70.0	77.5	85.0	92.5	100	115	130	145
26	33.8	37.7	41.6	46.8	49.4	57.2	65.0	72.8	80.6	88.4	96.2	104	119.6	135.2	150.8
27	35.1	39.2	43.2	48.6	51.3	59.4	67.5	75.6	83.7	91.8	99.9	108	124.2	140.4	156.6
28	36.4	40.6	44.8	50.4	53.2	61.6	70.	78.4	86.8	95.2	103.6	112	128.8	145.6	162.4
29	37.7	42.1	46.4	52.2	55.1	63.8	72.5	81.2	89.9	98.6	107.3	116	133.4	150.8	168.2
30	39.	43.5	48.0	54.	57.0	66.0	75.0	84.0	93.0	102.0	111.0	120	138	156	174
31	40.3	45.0	49.6	55.8	58.9	68.2	77.5	86.8	96.1	105.4	114.7	124	142.6	161.2	179.8
32	41.6	46.4	51.2	57.6	60.8	70.4	80.0	89.6	99.2	108.8	118.4	128	147.2	166.4	185.6
33	42.9	47.9	52.8	59.4	62.7	72.6	82.5	92.4	102.3	112.2	122.1	132	151.8	171.6	191.4
34	44.2	49.3	54.4	61.2	64.6	74.8	85.0	95.2	105.4	115.6	125.8	136	156.4	176.8	197.2
35	45.5	50.8	56.0	63.0	66.5	77.0	87.5	98.0	108.5	119.0	129.5	140	161	182	203
36	46.8	52.2	57.6	64.8	68.4	79.2	90.0	100.8	111.6	122.4	133.2	144	165.6	187.2	208.8
37	48.1	53.7	59.2	66.6	70.3	81.4	92.5	103.6	114.7	125.8	136.9	148	170.2	192.4	214.6
38	49.4	55.1	60.8	68.4	72.2	83.6	95.0	106.4	117.8	129.2	140.6	152	174.8	197.6	220.4
39	50.7	56.6	62.4	70.2	74.1	85.8	97.5	109.2	120.9	132.6	144.3	156	179.4	202.8	226.2
40	52	58.	64.0	72.0	76.0	88.0	100.	112.0	124.0	136.	148.0	160	184	208	232

CONSUMPTION RATE AT SURFACE (PSI PER MINUTE)

268

no-decompression limits and repetitive group designation table for no-decompression air dives

Depth (feet)	No-decompression limits (min)	A	B	C	D	E	F	G	H	I	J	K	L	M	N	O
10		60	120	210	300											
15		35	70	110	160	225	350									
20		25	50	75	100	135	180	240	325							
25	(245)	20	35	55	75	100	125	160	195	245	315					
30	(205)	15	30	45	60	75	95	120	145	170	205	250	310			
35	(160) 310	5	15	25	40	50	60	80	100	120	140	160	190	220	270	310
40	(130) 200	5	15	25	30	40	50	70	80	100	110	130	150	170	200	
50	(70) 100		10	15	25	30	40	50	60	70	80	90	100			
60	(50) 60		10	15	20	25	30	40	50	55	60					
70	(40) 50			5	10	15	20	30	35	40	45	50				
80	(30) 40			5	10	15	20	25	30	35	40					
90	(25) 30			5	10	12	15	20	25	30						
100	(20) 25			5	7	10	15	20	22	25						
110	(15) 20				5	10	13	15	20							
120	(10) 15				5	10	12	15								
130	(5) 10				5	8	10									
140	10				5	7	10									

residual nitrogen timetable for repetitive air dives

*Dives following surface intervals of more than 12 hours are not repetitive dives. Use actual bottom times in the Standard Air Decompression Tables to compute decompression for such dives.

The red line and red numbers on the no-decompression limits table above provide recommended limits based on ultrasound studies. The U.S. Navy Dive Table limits are based on extremely physically fit young males. For added safety, stop at 10 feet for one to three minutes at the end of each no-decompression dive. This helps to deplete most or all small nitrogen bubbles.

The black line on the lower table denotes U.S. Navy no-decompression limits. All residual nitrogen times listed to the left of the line will require the use of the Standard Air Decompression Table to compute decompression times and depths.

Repetitive group at the beginning of the surface interval

Group																
A	0:10 / 12:00*															
B	0:10–2:10 / 2:11–12:00*															
C	0:10–1:39 / 1:40–2:49 / 2:50–12:00*															
D	0:10–1:09 / 1:10–2:38 / 2:39–5:48 / 5:49–12:00*															
E	0:10–0:54 / 0:55–1:57 / 1:58–3:22 / 3:23–6:32 / 6:33–12:00*															
F	0:10–0:45 / 0:46–1:29 / 1:30–2:28 / 2:29–3:57 / 3:58–7:05 / 7:06–12:00*															
G	0:10–0:40 / 0:41–1:15 / 1:16–1:59 / 2:00–2:58 / 2:59–4:25 / 4:26–7:35 / 7:36–12:00*															
H	0:10–0:36 / 0:37–1:06 / 1:07–1:41 / 1:42–2:23 / 2:24–3:20 / 3:21–4:49 / 4:50–7:59 / 8:00–12:00*															
I	0:10–0:33 / 0:34–0:59 / 1:00–1:29 / 1:30–2:02 / 2:03–2:44 / 2:45–3:43 / 3:44–5:12 / 5:13–8:21 / 8:22–12:00*															
J	0:10–0:31 / 0:32–0:54 / 0:55–1:19 / 1:20–1:47 / 1:48–2:20 / 2:21–3:04 / 3:05–4:02 / 4:03–5:40 / 5:41–8:40 / 8:41–12:00*															
K	0:10–0:28 / 0:29–0:49 / 0:50–1:11 / 1:12–1:35 / 1:36–2:03 / 2:04–2:38 / 2:39–3:21 / 3:22–4:19 / 4:20–5:48 / 5:49–8:58 / 8:59–12:00*															
L	0:10–0:26 / 0:27–0:45 / 0:46–1:04 / 1:05–1:25 / 1:26–1:49 / 1:50–2:19 / 2:20–2:53 / 2:54–3:36 / 3:37–4:35 / 4:36–6:02 / 6:03–9:12 / 9:13–12:00*															
M	0:10–0:25 / 0:26–0:42 / 0:43–0:59 / 1:00–1:18 / 1:19–1:39 / 1:40–2:05 / 2:06–2:34 / 2:35–3:08 / 3:09–3:52 / 3:53–4:49 / 4:50–6:18 / 6:19–9:28 / 9:29–12:00*															
N	0:10–0:24 / 0:25–0:39 / 0:40–0:54 / 0:55–1:11 / 1:12–1:30 / 1:31–1:53 / 1:54–2:18 / 2:19–2:47 / 2:48–3:22 / 3:23–4:04 / 4:05–5:03 / 5:04–6:32 / 6:33–9:43 / 9:44–12:00*															
O	0:10–0:23 / 0:24–0:36 / 0:37–0:51 / 0:52–1:07 / 1:08–1:24 / 1:25–1:43 / 1:44–2:04 / 2:05–2:29 / 2:30–2:59 / 3:00–3:33 / 3:34–4:17 / 4:18–5:16 / 5:17–6:44 / 6:45–9:54 / 9:55–12:00*															
Z	0:10–0:22 / 0:23–0:34 / 0:35–0:48 / 0:49–1:02 / 1:03–1:18 / 1:19–1:36 / 1:37–1:55 / 1:56–2:17 / 2:18–2:42 / 2:43–3:10 / 3:11–3:45 / 3:46–4:29 / 4:30–5:27 / 5:28–6:56 / 6:57–10:05 / 10:06–12:00*															

NEW GROUP DESIGNATION / REPETITIVE DIVE DEPTH	Z	O	N	M	L	K	J	I	H	G	F	E	D	C	B	A
40	257	241	213	187	161	138	116	101	87	73	61	49	37	25	17	7
50	169	160	142	124	111	99	87	76	66	56	47	38	29	21	13	6
60	122	117	107	97	88	79	70	61	52	44	36	30	24	17	11	5
70	100	96	87	80	72	64	57	50	43	37	31	26	20	15	9	4
80	84	80	73	68	61	54	48	43	38	32	28	23	18	13	8	4
90	73	70	64	58	53	47	43	38	33	29	24	20	16	11	7	3
100	64	62	57	52	48	43	38	34	30	26	22	18	14	10	7	3
110	57	55	51	47	42	38	34	31	27	24	20	16	13	10	6	3
120	52	50	46	43	39	35	32	28	25	21	18	15	12	9	6	3
130	46	44	40	38	35	31	28	25	22	19	16	13	11	8	6	3
140	42	40	38	35	32	29	26	23	20	18	15	12	10	7	5	2

residual nitrogen times (minutes)

JEPPESEN

Unit	Abbreviation	Number of	Approximate U.S. equivalent		
Length					
myriameter	mym	10,000 meters	6.2 miles		
kilometer	km	1,000 meters	0.62 mile		
hectometer	hm	100 meters	109.36 yards		
dekameter	dam	10 meters	32.81 feet		
meter	m	1 meters	39.37 inches		
decimeter	dm	0.1 meters	3.94 inches		
centimeter	cm	0.01 meters	0.39 inch		
millimeter	mm	0.001 meters	0.04 inch		
Area					
square kilometer	sq km or km^2	1,000,000 sq. meters	0.3861 square mile		
hectare	ha	10,000 sq. meters	2.47 acres		
arc	a	100 sq. meters	119.60 square yards		
centare	ca	1 sq. meters	10.76 square feet		
square centimeter	sq cm or cm^2	0.0001 sq. meters	0.155 square inch		
Volume					
dekastere	das	10 cubic meters	13.10 cubic yards		
stere	s	1 cubic meters	1.31 cubic yards		
decistere	ds	0.10 cubic meters	3.53 cubic feet		
cubic centimeter	cu cm or cm' also cc	0.000001 cubic meters	0.061 cubic inch		
Capacity			CUBIC	DRY	LIQUID
kiloliter	kl	1,000 liters	1.31 cubic yards		
hectoliter	hl	100 liters	3.53 cubic feet	2.84 bushels	
dekaliter	dal	10 liters	0.35 cubic foot	1.14 pecks	2.64 gallons
liter	l	1 liters	61.02 cubic inches	0.908 quart	1.057 quarts
deciliter	dl	0.10 liters	6.1 cubic inches	0.18 pint	0.21 pint
centiliter	cl	0.01 liters	0.6 cubic inch		0.338 fluidounce
milliliter	ml	0.001 liters	0.06 cubic inch		0.27 fluidram

CONVERSION FACTORS

To convert			Multiply by
Length			
cm	to	inches	0.394
meters		feet	3.28
kilometers		nautical miles	0.540
inches	to	cm	2.54
feet		meters	0.3048
nautical miles		kilometers	1.853
Area			
cm^2	to	$inches^2$	0.155
$meters^2$		$feet^2$	10.76
$kilometers^2$		$miles^2$	0.386
$inches^2$	to	cm^2	6.45
$feet^2$		$meters^2$	0.093
$miles^2$		$kilometers^2$	0.3861
Volume and Capacity			
cc or ml	to	cu. inches	0.061
cu. meters		cu. feet	35.31
liters		cu. inches	61.02
liters		cu. feet	0.035
liters		fluid oz	33.81
liters		quarts	1.057
cu. inches	to	cc or ml	16.39
cu. feet		cu. meters	0.0283
quarts		liters	0.946
Weight			
grams	to	ounces	0.035
kilograms		pounds	2.205
ounces	to	grams	28.35
pounds		kilograms	0.454
Temperature			
°C	to	°F	9/5 then add 32
°F		°C	5/9 after subtracting 32
Pressure			
pounds per sq. in.	to	kg/cm^2	0.0703
pounds per sq. in.		cm of Hg	5.17
pounds per sq. in.		ft. of seawater	2.18
feet of seawater		psi	0.445

U.S. WEIGHTS AND MEASURES

Unit	Abbreviation or symbol	U.S. equivalent	Approximate metric equivalent
Length			
mile	mi	5280 feet, 320 rods, 1760 yards	1,609 kilometers
rod	rd	5.50 yards, 16.5 feet	5.029 meters
yard	yd	3 feet, 36 inches	0.914 meters
foot	ft or '	12 inches, 0.333 yards	30.480 centimeters
inch	in or "	0.083 feet, 0.027 yards	2.540 centimeters
Area			
square mile	sq mi or mi^2	640 acres, 102,400 square rods	2,590 square kilometers
acre		4840 square yards, 43,560 square feet	0.405 hectares, 4047 square meters
square rod	sq rd or rd^2	30.25 square yards, 0.006 acres	25.293 square meters
square yard	sq yd or yd^2	1296 square inches, 9 square feet	0.836 square meters
square foot	sq ft or ft^2	144 square inches, 0.111 square yards	0.093 square meters
square inch	sq in or in^2	0.007 square feet, 0.00077 square yards	6.451 square centimeters
Volume			
cubic yard	cu yd or yd^3	27 cubic feet, 46,656 cubic inches	0.765 cubic meters
cubic foot	cu ft or ft^3	1728 cubic inches, 0.0370 cubic yards	0.028 cubic meters
cubic inch	cu in or in^3	0.00058 cubic feet, 0.000021 cubic yards	16.387 cubic centimeters
Capacity		U.S. liquid measure	
gallon	gal	4 quarts (231 cubic inches)	3.785 liters
quart	qt	2 pints (57.75 cubic inches)	0.946 liters
pint	pt	4 gills (28.875 cubic inches)	0.473 liters
gill	gi	4 fluidounces (7.218 cubic inches)	118.291 milliliters
fluidounce	fl oz	8 fluidrams (1.804 cubic inches)	29.573 milliliters
fluidram	fl dr	60 minims (0.225 cubic inches)	3.696 milliliters
minim	min	1/00 fluidram (0.003759 cubic inches)	0.061610 milliliters

U.S. WEIGHTS AND MEASURES—cont'd

Unit	Abbreviation or symbol	U.S. equivalent	Approximate metric equivalent
Weight			
		Avoirdupois	
ton		20 short hundred-	
short ton		weight, 2000 pounds	0.907 metric tons
long ton		20 long hundredweight,	1.016 metric tons
		2240 pounds	
hundredweight	cwt		
short hundredweight		100 pounds, 0.05 short	45.159 kilograms
		tons	
long hundredweight		112 pounds, 0.05 long	50.802 kilograms
		tons	
pound	lb	16 ounces, 7000 grains	0.453 kilograms
ounce	ox	16 drams, 437.5 grains	28.349 grams
dram	dr	27.343 grains, 0.0625	1.771 grams
		ounces	
grain	gr	0.036 drams, 0.002285	0.0648 grams
		ounces	
		Troy	
pound	lb t	12 ounces, 240 penny-	0.373 kilograms
		weight, 5760 grains	
ounce	oz t	20 pennyweight, 480	31.103 grams
		grains	
pennyweight	dwt also pwt	24 grains, 0.05 ounces	1.555 grams
grain	gr	0.042 pennyweight,	0.0648 grams
		0.002083 ounces	

LOCATING YOUR NEAREST RECOMPRESSION CHAMBER

The following numbers may be called 24 hours a day, 7 days a week. Physicians are on call and consultation can be provided on air embolism or decompression sickness cases. Each maintains a world-wide listing of recompression chambers.

Divers Alert Network
DAN
919-684-8111

U.S. Navy Experimental Diving Unit
EDU Duty Phone
904-234-4353

EQUIPMENT CHECK LIST

Diving equipment

_____ Swim suit
_____ Mask
_____ Snorkel and snorkel keeper
_____ Fins
_____ Wet or dry suit
_____ Jacket
_____ Booties
_____ Gloves
_____ Pants
_____ Vest
_____ Hood
_____ Weight belt and weights
_____ Buoyancy compensator
_____ Full tank
_____ Regulator
_____ SPG
_____ Watch
_____ Depth gauge
_____ Compass
_____ Decompression tables
_____ Diver's flag and float
_____ Ascent/descent line and weight
_____ Whistle
_____ Knife
_____ Logbook and pencils
_____ Gear bag

Specialty items

_____ Diving computer
_____ Thermometer
_____ Emergency flare
_____ Dive light and batteries
_____ Slate and pencil
_____ Safety line (200 feet minimum)
_____ Buddy line
_____ Alternate air source

_____ Lift bag
_____ Photography equipment
_____ Strobe
_____ Camera
_____ Film
_____ Housing
_____ Batteries
_____ Spearfishing gear
_____ Speargun
_____ Game bag
_____ Fishing license

Spare parts and repair kit

_____ Mask strap and buckle
_____ Fin strap and buckle
_____ "O" rings
_____ Regulator high-pressure plug
_____ Silicone spray/grease
_____ Wet suit cement
_____ Sewing repair kit
_____ Extra mask lens
_____ Waterproof plastic tape
_____ Pliers/wrench/diver's tool
_____ Small knife
_____ BC repair patches

_____ **Other items**
_____ Dry clothes
_____ Towels
_____ Food and drinking water
_____ Sunglasses
_____ Suntan lotion
_____ Logbook
_____ Certification card
_____ Marine life identification guide

FIRST AID KIT COMPONENTS

_____ Utility shears
_____ Pocket mask with case
_____ Small flashlight with batteries
_____ Malleable, reusable splint
_____ 3-, 4-, and 6-inch conforming
bandage
_____ 4 × 4 inch dressings
_____ Multitrauma dressing
_____ Triangular bandages
_____ 3 inch hypoallergenic tape
_____ 1 inch BandAids
_____ Burn dressings
_____ Cold packs
_____ Hot packs
_____ Disposable blanket for hypother-
mia
_____ Oral glucose

_____ Sterile sodium chloride solution
(1 L minimum)
_____ Isopropyl alcohol
_____ Ammonia solution
_____ Acetic acid solution
_____ Antibiotic ointment
_____ Corticosteroid anti-inflammatory
ointment
_____ Oral diphenhydramine (Benadryl)
_____ Nonaspirin pain reliever
_____ Aspirin
_____ Motion sickness medication
_____ Sunblocker
_____ Shaving cream
_____ Disposable razors
_____ Cleansing towelettes

Index

A

Accidents
  environmental conditions of, 194
  first aid for, 219
Age, and physical conditioning, 176
Air bag bladder, 15
Air consumption
  in deep diving, 225-227
  factors influencing, 225-226
  formula and table for, 265-266
  table for at depth, 268
Air dump valve, 15-16
Air purity standards, 264
Air supply
  problems with, 178
  reduced levels of and stress, 188
  surface-supplied, 61-62
Air termination point, 149-150
Alcohol
  and decompression sickness, 243
  and deep diving, 230-231
Algae, turbidity caused by, 156
Alpha flag, 97
Alternate inflation regulator, 64-65
Anchor, 94
  handling of, 105
  location of, 145f
  true course to, 144f
Anchor line, following down, 237
Animals. *See also* Life forms
  active at night, 165-166, 172
  threat from, 177, 220
Archimedes principle, 264
Artifacts, collection of in turbid water,
    164-165
Ascent, 112
  air supply and, 178-179
  buddy-breathing, 188
  buoyancy during, 189
  in deep diving, 238-239
  direction control in, 163
    at night, 171
  emergency, 188
  rate of, 163, 238
  in rescue of unconscious diver, 204-206
  safety stop in, 239
  slow, 39
Ascent lines, in direction control, 161
Audible reserve, 29

B

Back-roll entry, 118
Backpack buoyancy compensator, 16-18, 19f
  maintenance of, 20
  and tank, 18-19
Balance, sensations used to maintain, 159
Balance organs, 159-160
BC. *See* Buoyancy compensator
Beach
  assessing conditions of, 84
  landing on, 119
Beach diving, 81-83
  currents in, 84-85
  entries and exits in, 85-90
  equipment for, 82
  on high-land low-impact beaches, 84
  planning of, 84
Behavioral toxicity, 229, 260
Bilge, 94
Bioluminescence, 165
Bleeding, first aid for, 219
Board-mounted compass, 129f, 130
Boat, 92-93
  beach landing of, 119
  diving techniques for on small boat, 117-119
  propellers of, 177
  reentry techniques for on small boat, 118
  returning to, 111-114
  selection of, 116-119
  set-up for deep dive, 234-236
  types and parts of, 94-95
Boat diving, 91-93
  advantages of, 108
  boat owner-operator Coast Guard
    requirements, 115-116
  checklist for, 99f
  Coast Guard requirements for, 96-99
  commercial, 96
  dive boats for, 94-95
  equipment for, 100-101
  fitness for, 101-102
  forms of, 108-111
  general conduct in, 102-103
  at night, 171
  planning of, 102
  post-dive procedures in, 114-115
  preparation for, 100-102, 105-108
  returning to boat in, 111-114
  selection of boat for, 116-117